Dee & D'Andra Simmons

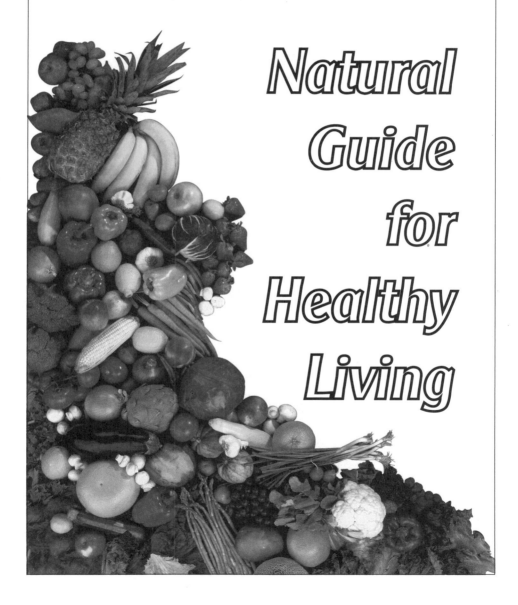

Natural Guide for Healthy Living

Natural Guide for Healthy Living

Dedication

This book is dedicated to our dear and loving husbands, Glenn and David. Without their continued support, encouragement, and unconditional love, this collaboration would have never been possible. Without us they would be hopeless victims of the SAD (Standard American Diet).

We thank them for never tiring of our dreams and ambitions, and especially for keeping us focused. They are our heroes!

Dee and D'Andra

Dee & D'Andra Simmons Natural Guide for Healthy Living
Published by Dee Simmons

This book is not intended to provide medical advice or to take the place of medical advice and treatment from your personal physician. Readers are advised to consult their own doctors or other qualified health professionals regarding the treatment of their medical problems. Neither the publisher nor the author takes any responsibility for any possible consequences from any treatment, action or application of medicine, supplement, herb or preparation to any person reading or following the information in this book. If readers are taking prescription medications, again, they should consult with their physicians and not take themselves off medicines to start a supplementation or nutrition program without the proper supervision of a physician.

Printed in the United States of America

Table of Contents

Table of Contents

Table of Contents

Chapter Fifteen: Anti-Aging (continued)

Chapter Sixteen
Skin Care **259**

Natural Guide for Healthy Living

Dee and D'Andra Simmons
Natural Guide for Healthy Living

Y ou may be wealthy. You may be brilliant. You may be famous. You may be successful. But if you do not have good health, not one of these things matters. You cannot enjoy your life to the fullest if you are not well. Dee Simmons discovered this first hand when she was diagnosed with cancer in 1987. She then embarked on a journey of faith, learning, and empowerment that saw her cancer healed and led to her realization of the importance of being proactive in one's health and wellness. D'Andra Simmons-Manges, Dee's daughter, has lost her grandmother to cancer and has watched both her aunt and mother fight the disease.

Since her cancer diagnosis and subsequent remission, Dee has spent years traveling to meet with some of the world's greatest experts in the areas of natural and alternative healthcare. In developing her own line of healthcare supplements, she has interviewed the world's finest chemists and has been blessed to have spent time with some of the foremost authorities on nutrition and nutritional supplements. She wants you to benefit from what she has learned.

The medical profession is now acknowledging the positive effects of good nutrition, a healthy lifestyle, and a joyous outlook. What used to be regarded by medical professionals as "junk science" is now a part of treatment protocol for people suffering from a large number of diseases. Many hospitals currently offer complementary treatments to augment traditional therapies. Dee and D'Andra firmly believe in using the best of science and the best of nature to combat disease and to stay healthy.

How often do you now hear that proper nutrition, weight loss, and stress reduction will prevent debilitating diseases? Constantly! Did you know that you can achieve these goals naturally and with very little effort? It simply takes knowledge and guidance. Dee wants to spare you the disease she experienced and to offer you the benefit of all she has learned in her efforts to prevent cancer from recurring.

A world traveler and Bush Administration appointee, D'Andra left Washington to work with her mother. An expert on skin care, she offers important advice on keeping your skin fresh and young even while living a hectic lifestyle. D'Andra stresses the importance of starting the battle early against disease and aging. Dee and D'Andra want you to live each and every day feeling and looking your best so you can appreciate all the blessings this life has to offer.

Francisco Contreras, M.D.

A Message From Dee

Getting healthy and staying healthy takes motivation. What motivates one person may not be a jump-start for another. But let's face it. All of us want to feel and look our best. And as we age, the motivation becomes stronger because it takes more effort to stay well and avoid the negative aspects of aging. For many, the mirror is the motivation, and the truth is, if you are healthy, the mirror will reflect it. What motivated me to take charge of my health was a dramatic experience – the diagnosis of breast cancer in 1987.

After my diagnosis, I became determined to conquer the disease and to keep it from recurring. I was fortunate to have the resources to pursue my quest to learn everything I could about nutrition and its positive effects. I gave up a lucrative fashion business to virtually save my life. Fortunately Glenn, my husband, has been a generous and supportive partner in my endeavors.

My search introduced me to some very interesting places and people–some expected, such as nutrition laboratories and famous doctors, others very surprising, such as jungle huts and whacky practitioners. I was driven to educate myself and to examine all the possibilities that science and nature have to offer in the fight against disease. Every single doctor, chemist, and practitioner agreed on one thing: nutrition plays a vital role in our overall health and well-being. Consequently, my focus became directed to nutrition, specifically the study of green foods.

The positive effects of green foods on our immune systems are unquestionable; and, since my motivation was to boost my immune system to stave off a recurrence of cancer, I searched for the best green food I could find and found it. I developed my own! So effective was what I called **Green Miracle** that I began to share it with family and friends who immediately felt the same positive effects I had been describing: a boost in energy levels, overall better health with fewer colds and viruses, and a general feeling of well-being. **Green Miracle** became the cornerstone of Ultimate Living International, my now ten year old nutritional company.

It should not take a life-threatening illness to motivate you to take charge of your health. When cancer appeared, I was a complete workaholic, working in a competitive and pressure-filled environment, eating on the run, eating a high fat diet, driving my body to the limit, and operating most of the time on far too little rest. If this sounds familiar, take a hard look at how your lifestyle is affecting your health and benefit from my experience. Slow down, improve your eating habits, and get rest. These three lifestyle changes alone can dramatically improve your odds against disease.

Five years after I was diagnosed with cancer my dear mother passed away from pancreatic cancer. Not only did I become more motivated than ever to combat this scourge, but my life also took on a new mission—to educate others on the importance, the necessity, of taking charge of your health and that of your family. In the years following my mother's death, my company has developed a family of pure, natural, and effective nutritional products, and I spend as much time as possible speaking to individuals and groups in an effort to pass along my knowledge on the subject of nutrition.

Five years ago, my only sister was diagnosed with breast cancer and was given a poor prognosis. We went to battle together. She had excellent medical care and took advantage of natural therapies as well. She increased her consumption of green foods and took supplements where appropriate. I counseled with her every step of the way. The combination of science and nature gave her the best chance for a good outcome, and, thankfully, today she is cancer-free.

It is inspirational to see great outcomes. Positive experiences can be just as life-changing as negative ones. Seeing my sister feel well throughout her treatment, largely due to her good nutrition, has re-energized my mission to teach nutrition and a healthy lifestyle and, of course, the virtues of green foods whenever and wherever people will listen.

My hopes, like those of most parents, lie with my daughter. In a family fraught with cancer, my greatest motivation is to see her remain free of the disease. She has recently returned from working with the Bush Administration in Washington, D.C., to join my company and our mission.

I guess it is easy to see that my biggest motivator has been my own family. I want to pass my motivation and my knowledge on to you. I believe that it is never too late to take charge of your health and that of your loved ones!

For me, however, faith has also been an essential element. Throughout my life I have been buoyed by faith, and faith has been shown to have extraordinary effects on disease prevention and cure, even longevity. Faith has been the cornerstone of my personal and business life and is the guiding factor that above all else has enabled me to be healed, to achieve my goals, and to pass on what I have learned to others.

Dee Simmons

A Message from D'Andra

It was March 1987, and I was anticipating heading off to college in Virginia and spending the next four years away from my family and my Texas home. This was to be my first big adventure in growing up. Little did I know that my birthday, March 15, would not only mark my transition from teenager to adulthood, but would be forever remembered as a dark time in my life. On my birthday, my mother lay in a hospital bed after undergoing a modified radical mastectomy and reconstruction that left us all perplexed and bewildered.

My mother had always been the picture of health. She was tall, thin, a former model, and had never even had a cold in her life, much less cancer! At that time, cancer was not much talked about. It was known as the big "C," and I thought that the only people who contracted it were older people, people who smoked, and those who chose to live unhealthy lives. So why was this happening to my mom, a woman who had never held a cigarette in her life and who very rarely even had a glass of wine? We always had vegetables with dinner, and she made certain our meals were balanced according to the guidelines of the nutritional food pyramid. How could she be a victim of cancer?

As a result of her cancer, my mother became interested in alternative health and nutrition. She stunned her doctors by choosing not to follow up her mastectomy with chemotherapy and radiation. Instead, she chose to take her chances with what at that time was a mysterious and almost unknown phenomenon–the world of holistic nutrition, herbology, and alternative therapies.

The next few years of my mother's life were spent traveling the world with my father, learning everything from the "how to" of juicing to the benefits of herbal remedies and the importance of detoxification. She even experimented with live cell therapy and laetrile treatments. As my mother gained knowledge, she chose to do away with every nutritional concept she had previously learned. In the end, she changed my beliefs about nutrition as well. I was not only her daughter but also her personal project and, more often than not, her guinea pig. I tried every green food, every herbal potion, every detoxification program, and I was part of each new discovery as we both searched for knowledge and the answer to staying healthy and cancer free.

A lot has transpired in eighteen years. Five years after my mother's diagnosis, my grandmother was diagnosed with pancreatic cancer and died after one month. A month does not provide much time to say goodbye to someone who has meant so much in your life. Knowing that there is nothing you can do even though you are armed with a wealth of knowledge is even more frightening than the realization of a certain death. Five years later my grandfather was diagnosed with prostate and bone cancer. We could not save him either, and this time I watched the cancer ravage his body and mind, causing him excruciating pain. Both of my grandparents had lived exemplary lives. They did not drink or smoke, and they were upstanding members of their church and community. I learned that cancer is not a respecter of persons.

In spite of what has happened to many members of my family, I do have hope. Eighteen years after my mother's cancer diagnosis, I am happy to report that she remains cancer free. In addition, her sister, who was diagnosed with breast cancer five years ago, is still with us, the first cancer survivor in our family since my mother. She is our family's second miracle in eighteen years, and we believe this is partially due to the holistic therapies and regimen she has followed under my mother's guidance. I remain the only woman on my mother's side of the family who has not fallen victim to cancer. My real test will be these next ten to fifteen years as I struggle to keep myself purged of free radicals and my immune system ready to battle invasive carcinogens.

My mother's quest to save her own life has become a mission to save others as well, and her quest has also become mine. After years of serving as a spokesperson for a nutritional company and counseling cancer patients who came to her for advice, my mother decided to start her own nutrition and skin care company, Ultimate Living International, Inc. I joined her company last year in the hope that I, like my mother, can make a difference in people's health. I, too, have become a student of nutrition with my mother still my best teacher. A newlywed, I hope to instill in my family the same good health habits that she has for so long instilled in me.

I am particularly interested in skin care. Interest in anti-aging is growing as doctors and researchers look for more ways to keep us young. In recent years, experts have connected nutrition not only with good health but also with anti-aging.

In her sixties and even as a cancer-survivor, Mother looks fabulous! A devotee to green foods and natural supplements, she created a skin care division of our company to feed the body's largest organ–skin. Dee Simmons Skin Care products have no harmful chemicals and are made with the purest, most effective ingredients available.

We are constantly updating and upgrading our skin care line to include the latest breakthroughs in anti-aging. This means meeting regularly with some of the world's leading authorities, all of whom agree on the things I have long learned from my mother–the importance of a healthy lifestyle and good nutrition for staying well and looking your best.

Now in my mid-thirties, I also know the importance of taking good care of my skin to stave off the signs of aging and to keep that healthy glow that comes with great nutrition and skin care. I have found that looking your very best comes naturally when you are in optimum health.

D'Andra Simmons

- *Did you know there are foods that can actually strengthen the immune system?*

- *If you or a loved-one is being treated for cancer, did you know that there are foods that can actually diminish the side effects of cancer treatment?*

- *New dietary guidelines are confusing. How many fruits and vegetables do we need each day? Which are best? What constitutes a serving?*

- *Thousands of anti-aging products are on the market. What works? What doesn't?*

- *Many of you are already doing great things for your health–walking, lifting free weights, watching your diet– but did you know there are foods and supplements that can augment your efforts?*

Let Dee and D'Andra answer your questions in the following pages.

*Our greatest hope is that you will
use the information contained on these pages
to guide you and your loved-ones towards
healthy living–naturally!*

Are You Ready to Feel Better?

Since you have read this far it is apparent that you are endeavoring to take charge of your health. The information offered on these pages is designed to provide you with the tools you need to combat the most common ailments naturally. If you are already suffering from a chronic illness, this book will help you do the most you can to stay well while battling your disorder. It is now known that diet, obesity, stress, and many other factors that can be controlled definitely contribute to such illnesses as cancer, diabetes, and heart disease. It is never too late to revise our behavior and change our lifestyle to lessen our odds of becoming ill.

What Are You Eating?

Remember, the foods discussed in this book should always be as close to whole, natural, unrefined, and untreated as possible. Organic is always best when available. When we talk about water, filtered water is best, especially when filtered through the reverse osmosis process. Let's face it! Our environment is not user-friendly. We have to combat the ill-effects of toxins and chemicals by making the right choices when we are at the grocery store.

What's Eating You?

Every one of the common ailments discussed in this book is worsened by stress. Did you know that stress can even inhibit your ability to lose weight? We will discuss foods that comfort you and activities that calm you—nature's tranquilizers.

Overcoming Illness

The answer to overcoming illness lies in your immune system. The secret to getting well and staying well lies there. Get ready to learn the best methods for strengthening your body's ability to ward off disease and to overcome ill-health when it happens.

Ready, Set

As you read on, you will see that optimizing your health is dependent upon several components and that you cannot attain optimum wellness unless each is addressed. Your mental state may be the single most important force in your getting well and staying well. Your mind has control over your actions and your body so get ready to develop a healthy, positive mind-set. Your body relies on you to take care of it. You are solely responsible for the care of your health. Get ready to take charge! If you are suffering from a chronic illness, get ready to arm yourself with nature's weapons to fight your malady.

Although the spiritual aspects of your life are your individual choice, research shows definitively that persons with strong faith by and large are healthier and more apt to overcome serious illness than those without faith. Statistics regarding the power of prayer are undeniable. Strengthening your faith is a major factor in strengthening your immune system.

Go!

Let's get moving toward good health.

Chapter One

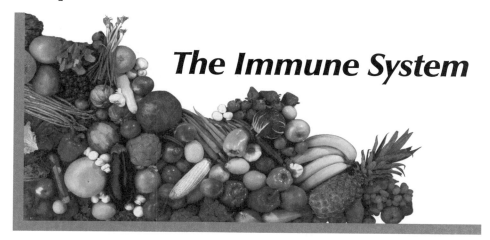

The Immune System

T he immune system is where good health begins and, unfortunately, ends. The good news is that every year we learn more and more about keeping our immune systems strong.

If you are fortunate to be in good health, no doubt you want to maximize your odds of staying healthy. If you have overcome an illness, you want to make certain that it does not recur. The secret of both rests solely under the control of your immune system. It is the immune system that protects the body from bacteria, viruses, fungi, and many other harmful substances.

Today our immune systems are overworked and overtaxed. Our environment, loaded with stress, toxins, bacteria, and viruses, keeps our immune systems constantly working overtime. Toxins in food and the environment, poor diet, and, of course, ubiquitous stress can dramatically weaken the immune system. Add self-imposed habits such as smoking, alcohol consumption, poor diet, and lack of rest, and the whole scenario is a recipe for illness.

Believe it or not, the study of the immune system is relatively recent. In the late eighteenth century, Edward Jenner discovered that humans could be protected from smallpox by inoculation with cowpox, a relative of the smallpox virus. The principle of this vaccination is that a vaccinated individual develops a specific immune response to cowpox, thus receiving protection from smallpox. This early research made clear the critical role that the immune system and its antibodies can play in the treatment and prevention of disease. In 1979, smallpox became the first human disease to be completely eradicated.

Many current cancer studies are focusing on the immune system. In the future, selective immune responses may become useful therapeutic tools in the fight against cancer. A promising new approach to treating cancer is to try to generate an immune response against the cancer itself by vaccinating a patient with his/her own cancer cells or with tumor extracts.

By gaining understanding of the workings of the immune system and finding ways to strengthen its natural ability to fight disease, immunologists have developed a new approach to cancer treatment. Immunotherapy is beginning to show much promise in the field of cancer-care and other major diseases.

While the immune system is responsible for protecting us against major illness, it also shoulders the responsibility of defending us from everyday sicknesses such as colds, viruses, and infections from minor injuries and the like. If you take good care of your immune system, it will respond by taking better care of you.

Your Bodyguard

The immune system is amazing! It is designed to defend you against bacteria, microbes, viruses, toxins, and parasites. Think about the environment and its complex makeup of all of those things. We are exposed to literally millions of immune system enemies everyday, including poor nutrition, x-rays, alcohol, cigarette smoke, and other pollutants. If our immune system is working in good order, our bodies can resist disease, infection, even poisoning. Yet we seldom think about our immune systems until they fail us. We get a cold, we catch the flu, or, worse, we contract a serious illness such as cancer.

The immune system will also make you take notice when it goes astray. Allergies, for example, are the result of the immune system overreacting to certain things that do not bother most people. Diabetes is caused by the immune system attacking and destroying cells in the pancreas. People with rheumatoid arthritis have a disease caused by the immune system attacking the joints.

There are, in fact, a number of diseases that are the result of the immune system going awry. And while the exact cause of these occurrences—known as autoimmune responses—may not be known, we do know that strengthening the immune system is the single best way to avoid these problems as well as other diseases.

Your skin is also a significant part of the immune system. It acts as the body's armor, but, at the same time, our orifices (nose, mouth, eyes) are opportune places for germs to enter the body. The amazing immune system is ready for those invaders, too. Our tears, even mucus, contain an enzyme that breaks down bacterial cell walls. Our nasal passages, lungs, throat, and skin are lined with mast cells that kill bacteria. So invaders have to pass through a myriad of defense systems. Once germs do get in, they have to deal with other defenses, for instance the lymphatic system which is designed to recognize and dispose of germs and bacteria. Here's the problem. Like our blood, lymph travels through our system in a path, but, unlike our blood, lymph is not under pressure. Rather, it oozes through our bodies, relying on our movements to get it going. Immune system cells are produced by the thymus gland, the spleen, and other organs. They are carried throughout the body by the lazy lymphatic system. One of the benefits of regular exercise is getting the lymph system moving. The thymus, the spleen, bone marrow, white blood cells, certain proteins, and hormones all work to rid the body of germs and foreign invaders.

It boggles the mind to think of the complexity of the system that we rely upon to stay well–to stay alive.

Antioxidants to the Rescue

The enemies to the immune system are free radicals. Free radicals exist everywhere in the present environment, and we now know that they are responsible for damaging healthy cells and causing debilitating diseases such as cancer and heart disease. Free radicals "stalk" stable molecules to "steal" their electrons. When the "attacked" molecule loses its electron, it becomes a free radical itself. This is the start of a chain reaction. Once started, the process can escalate, finally resulting in the disruption of a living cell. Some free radicals occur normally during metabolism, and occasionally the immune system's cells create them to neutralize viruses and bacteria. However, environmental factors such as pollution, radiation, cigarette smoke, and herbicides generate free radicals continuously.

Fortunately, there are substances that can destroy free radicals– **antioxidants**. Normally the body can handle free radicals, but if antioxidants are unavailable, or if the free-radical production becomes excessive, damage can occur. Of particular importance is that free radical damage increases with age. Antioxidants can help offset the damage, and they are available to us in many of the foods we eat (or should eat).

Vitamin C

Vitamin C is the big dog of antioxidants. Vitamin C is a real immune system booster. As a matter of fact, diets rich in vitamin C are believed to reduce the risk of breast, colorectal, stomach, and prostate cancers. The best sources of vitamin C are organic fruits and vegetables such as citrus fruits, green peppers, cantaloupes, broccoli, cranberries, and papaya. The daily requirement is 60 mg (one medium-size orange); however, that is very minimal. Five hundred milligrams a day is much better. At times we have even taken 1,000 to 5,000 mg per day in an effort to fight an oncoming cold or virus.

Studies have found that vitamin C may:

- ○ *Contribute to healthy bones*
- ○ *Help prevent periodontal disease*
- ○ *Aid in healing wounds*
- ○ *Combat inflammation and pain*
- ○ *Aid iron absorption*
- ○ *Break down histamine*
- ○ *Offer potent antioxidant protection*
- ○ *Protect lung function*
- ○ *Maintain cognition in the elderly*

Since our bodies do not produce vitamin C, it is important that we derive it from other sources. The ideal way is to eat organic fruits and vegetables rich in vitamin C.

Fruits containing Vitamin C include:

Berries	**Oranges**
Cantaloupe	**Papayas**
Grapefruit	**Peaches**
Guava	**Persimmons**
Lemons	**Pineapples**
Limes	**Strawberries (fresh)**
Mangoes	**Tangerines**

Good vegetable sources of Vitamin C are:

Alfalfa	Lettuce
Asparagus	Mustard greens
Avocados	Onions
Beet greens	Potatoes
Broccoli	Radishes
Brussel sprouts	Spinach
Cabbage	Sweet potatoes
Collards	Swiss chard
Dandelion greens	Tomatoes
Green and red bell peppers	Turnip greens
Green peas	Watercress
Kale	

Vitamin A

Vitamin A is a family of fat-soluble vitamins. Retinol is one of the most active, or usable, forms of vitamin A, and it is found in animal foods such as liver and eggs and in some fortified food products. Vitamin A helps regulate the immune system. The immune system helps prevent or fight off infections by making white blood cells that destroy harmful bacteria and viruses.

Vitamin A may help lymphocytes, a type of white blood cell that fights infections, function more effectively. Vitamin A is found in animal foods such as eggs, whole milk, and liver. Most fat free milk and dried nonfat milk solids sold in the U.S. are fortified with vitamin A to replace the vitamin A lost when the fat is removed. Fortified foods such as fortified breakfast cereals also provide vitamin A.

Some plant foods contain darkly colored pigments called provitamin A carotenoids that can be converted to vitamin A. In the U.S., a large percentage of the vitamin A that is consumed is provided by provitamin A carotenoids.

Vitamin A plays an important role in vision, bone growth, reproduction, cell division, and cell differentiation (the process by which a cell decides what it is going to become).

> *Important: Vitamin A can become toxic in larger doses unless it is taken in the form of beta carotene.*

Carotenoids

Carotenoids are antioxidants that help strengthen the immune system by producing lymphocytes. Lymphocytes are cells important in fighting infection. The best sources for carotenoids are the red, yellow, and orange fruits and vegetables such as carrots, tomatoes, cantaloupes, papaya, pumpkin, and leafy green foods.

The four important carotenoids are **beta-carotene, lycopene, lutein,** and **zeaxanthin**. Lutein and zeaxanthin are found in leafy greens such as kale and spinach. All of these provide excellent protection against disease.

Carotenoids also play an important potential role in human health by acting as biological antioxidants, protecting cells and tissues from the damaging effects of free radicals. Carotenoids are thought to protect the body from the damaging effects of the sun and may therefore play a critical role in the prevention of skin cancers. (See Chapter 8)

The Institute of Medicine (IOM) encourages consumption of carotenoid-rich fruits and vegetables for their health-promoting benefits.

Surveys suggest an association between diets rich in beta-carotene and vitamin A and a lower risk of some types of cancer. There is evidence that a higher intake of green and yellow vegetables or other food sources of beta-carotene and/or vitamin A may decrease the risk of lung cancer.

Beta-Carotene

Beta-carotene is probably the best known of the carotenoids, those red, orange, and yellow pigments that give color to many fruits and vegetables. The body converts beta-carotene into vitamin A, a nutrient first identified in the 1930s and now recognized as vital to the growth and development of the human body.

Beta-carotene is a provitamin A carotenoid that is more efficiently converted to retinol than other carotenoids. Dietary beta-carotene is obtained from a number of fruits and vegetables, such as carrots, spinach, peaches, apricots, and sweet potatoes.

As a potent immune system booster and a powerful antioxidant that counters the effects of cell-damaging molecules called free-radicals, beta-carotene has an important role to play in human health.

Consuming plenty of organic fruits and vegetables is an excellent way to supply your body with beta-carotene.

Lycopene

Lycopene is an antioxidant that has received a lot of attention from researchers in recent years. Lycopene is a pigment that gives vegetables and fruits, such as tomatoes, pink grapefruit, and watermelon, their red color. It also appears to have strong antioxidant capabilities. Several studies suggest that consumption of foods rich in lycopene is associated with a lower risk of prostate cancer (page 98) and cardiovascular disease.

In a 1995 Harvard University study conducted with 47,894 men, researchers found that eating ten or more servings a week of tomato products was associated with a reduced risk of prostate cancer by as much as 34 percent.

The protective effect of antioxidants on heart disease has been well documented. In a recently published study, men who had the highest amount of lycopene in their body fat were half as likely to suffer a heart attack as those with the least amount of lycopene in their body fat. Researchers have determined that the level of lycopene in body fat is an indicator of lycopene content in the diet.

Lycopene is not produced in the body, so you can only obtain its benefits by eating foods rich in lycopene. Tomato products, such as spaghetti sauce, tomato juice, ketchup, and pizza sauce are, by far, the major sources of lycopene in the typical American diet. In fact, these foods provide over 80 percent of the lycopene consumed in the U.S. Other fruits and vegetables such as watermelon and pink grapefruit also provide lycopene but in smaller amounts.

Lycopene is better absorbed by the body when it is consumed in processed tomato products rather than fresh tomatoes. The reason for this remains unclear. In one study lycopene was absorbed 2.5 times better from tomato paste than from fresh tomatoes. However, cooking fresh tomatoes with a little oil greatly increases lycopene absorption.

Bioflavonoids

Bioflavonoids are a group of phytonutrients that aid the immune system by protecting the cells of the body against environmental pollutants. Bioflavonoids also reduce cholesterol's ability to form plaque in arteries and lessen the formation of microscopic clots inside the arteries that can lead to heart attack and stroke.

Studies have shown that people who eat the most bioflavonoids have less cardiovascular disease. A diet that contains a wide variety of organic fruits and vegetables, at least six servings per day, will help you get the bioflavonoids needed to keep your immune system working efficiently.

Bioflavonoids and vitamin C are found in many of the same foods and the body metabolizes both of these in the same manner. Researchers have discovered that some of the functions with which vitamin C is credited are actually from the bioflavonoids.

Foods that are high in bioflavonoids include blueberries, apricots, blackberries, black currants, broccoli, cantaloupes, cherries, grapefruits, grapes, oranges, and lemons.

Disease Fighters

Vitamin E helps to slow the aging process. It also helps the body to fight bacteria and viruses. Research has found that vitamin E helps in the fight against heart disease and cancer. Whole grain foods and vegetable oils are great sources of this valuable vitamin, but supplements are almost always required in order to reach the daily minimum requirement. To be really effective, to help in the battle against cancer and heart disease, 400 mg is optimum. It's not difficult to get 30 to 60 milligrams every day of vitamin E from a diet rich in seeds, vegetable oils, and grains, but it's difficult for most people to consume more than 60 milligrams a day consistently through diet alone. Supplements may be necessary to get enough vitamin E to boost your immune system.

Vitamin E stimulates the production of natural killer cells, those that seek out and destroy germs and cancer cells. Vitamin E enhances the production of B-cells, the immune cells that produce antibodies that destroy bacteria. Vitamin E supplementation may also reverse some of the decline in immune response commonly seen in aging. Vitamin E has been implicated in lowering the risk of cardiovascular disease. In the Harvard School of Public Health study of 87,000 nurses, vitamin E supplementation was shown to cut the risk of heart attacks by fifty percent.

Selenium helps to increase the number of antibodies and encourages growth of immune cells. This mineral increases natural killer cells and mobilizes cancer-fighting cells. The best food sources of selenium are tuna, red snapper, whole grains, vegetables (depending on the selenium content of the soil in which they are grown), brown rice, egg yolks, cottage cheese, chicken (white meat), sunflower seeds, garlic, Brazil nuts, and lamb chops.

Zinc is a mineral essential to several immune-system functions. The immune system gains strength from minerals in order to synthesize proteins that make up all the cells of the body. Zinc helps with healing and may reduce infection while at the same time helping the body to produce antibodies. By helping to regulate the function of white blood cells, zinc can improve antibody responses to vaccines and cell-mediated immunity. Dietary sources of zinc are whole grains, lentils, chicken, almonds, and pumpkin seeds. Zinc is excellent to combat skin disorders, especially acne.

Acidophilus is a beneficial bacteria that inhabits the human digestive system. It is best known for assuring the return of normal body functions after a course of antibiotics by reintroducing friendly bacteria into the colon. It acts as a mild antibiotic, and regular use can replace the harmful bacteria in your colon. In women, acidophilus has been used to treat vaginal yeast infections.

Coenzyme-Q10 is made in the body and works with other enzymes to support bioenergetic functions. It also seems to act as a mild stimulant to the immune system and has been shown to help lower blood pressure and to enhance the pumping action and electrical function of the heart. It may also improve energy production in heart muscle cells.

Coenzyme Q10 is made naturally by the human body. It helps cells to produce energy, and it acts as an antioxidant. It has shown an ability to stimulate the immune system and to protect the heart from damage caused by certain chemotherapy drugs. Low blood levels of CoQ10 have been detected in patients with some types of cancer. Studies with CoQ10 have mostly focused on its role involving certain types of cardiovascular diseases, including congestive heart failure and hypertension. CoQ10 has also been evaluated for its positive effects on high cholesterol and diabetes. It is also an excellent remedy for gum and periodontal disease.

As a supplement, CoQ10 may help treat congestive heart failure and delay the progression of Parkinson's disease. It may also be useful in treating diseases including muscular dystrophy, AIDS, hypertension, and mitochondrial encephalomyopathies.

> **B complex *vitamins** play a role in nourishing the immune system.*

> **B-12** is an important nutrient for the immune system because it aids in the formation of red blood cells and antibodies. B-12 prevents anemia and is effective in restoring mental clarity.

> **Vitamin B-6** is involved in more body functions than any other nutrient and affects both mental and physical health. Carpal tunnel syndrome has been linked to B-6 deficiency.

> **Pantothenic acid** serves as a part of the coenzyme A which is essential for the production of energy, for the production of antibodies, and for the healthy maintenance of the central nervous system.

> **Folic acid** is necessary for the growth of all types of cells in the body, including white blood cells. It also takes part in the process of cell division and in the healthy growth of glands, including the

thymus. For women of child-bearing age, folic acid is imperative to sustain pregnancy and prevent birth defects.

The B complex vitamins have many functions, and it may be important to take extra B complex vitamins when you are undergoing a lot of stress. Prolonged stress will decrease the function of your immune system.

L-Cysteine is essential for the proper use of vitamin B-6 and serves as a part of the body's heavy metal detoxification system.

Iron fights infection and strengthens overall immunity. However, too much iron can be harmful, and a physician should be consulted before starting a program of using iron supplements. Meats, dried beans, and tofu are good sources of iron.

Echinacea is one of the most popular and effective herbal remedies for strengthening the immune system. Other immune system herbs are Siberian ginseng, goldenseal, astralagus, and horseradish root. But remember, before you take any herbal preparations, talk to your physician. A knowledgeable health food store can help you make herbal selections.

People with allergies need to be very cautious in taking herbal remedies. Individuals suffering with ragweed allergies, for instance, may be sensitive to echinacea. Echinacea stimulates the immune system and may also protect against infection and stimulate tissue repair and healing.

Alpha lipoic acid is one of the most effective antioxidants to fight free radicals and helps boost glutathione levels in the body. Glutathione is a protein found in our cells that is important for healthy immune system function.

Essential Fatty Acids

Essential fatty acids are important to the immune system because they reduce inflammation associated with allergic response by aiding in the production of prostaglandins that counter inflammation. Essential fatty acids are found in cold water fish, flaxseed, and flax oil.

A study found that children taking a half teaspoon of flax oil a day experienced fewer and less severe respiratory infections and fewer days of being absent from school. The Omega-3 fatty acids in flax oil and fatty fish (such as salmon, tuna, and mackerel) act as immune boosters by increasing the activity of phagocytes, the white blood cells that eat up bacteria. (Perhaps this is why grandmothers used to insist on a daily dose of unpalatable cod liver oil.) Essential fatty acids also protect the body against damage from over-reactions to infection.

> **This may surprise you:**
> *Garlic is a healer. The flavorful member of the onion family is a powerful immune booster that stimulates the multiplication of infection-fighting white cells, boosts natural killer cell activity, and increases the efficiency of antibody production.*

When taking essential fatty acid supplements, such as flax or fish oils, take additional vitamin E, which acts together with essential fatty acids to boost the immune system. One way to get more Omega-3 fatty acids in your diet is to add one to three teaspoons of flax oil to a fruit and yogurt smoothie.

The immune-boosting properties of garlic seem to be due to its sulfur-containing compounds, such as allicin and sulfides. Garlic can also act as an antioxidant that reduces the build-up of free radicals in the bloodstream. Although the evidence is controversial, garlic may protect against cancer. Cultures with a garlic-rich diet have a lower incidence of intestinal cancer. Garlic may also play a part in getting rid of potential carcinogens and other toxic substances. It is also a heart-friendly food since it keeps platelets from sticking together and clogging tiny blood vessels.

Get in Your Immune System's Corner

In order to give your immune system a fighting chance, you need to make certain that you make a habit of doing the following:

- Hands down, the best way to prevent colds and flu is hand washing. Think about the points of entry for germs into your body. Wash your hands frequently, and do not put your hands in your eyes, nose, and mouth. If you receive an injury, wash it thoroughly with antibacterial soap and keep the wound clean. We have a friend who is a health correspondent for a major television network. He covers the flu season annually and tells us that every authority says the same thing, "Hand washing will eliminate a tremendous amount of colds and flu." How easy is that? Aren't a few bottles of anti-bacterial soaps and wipes better than a bout with the flu?

- Exercise regularly to keep your lymph system moving. There is no need to overdo it, but try to exercise moderately for thirty minutes at least five times a week. Remember, unlike our blood stream, the lymph system needs for us to help it circulate, so get off that couch and move.

- Eat a diet rich in antioxidants and take supplements to augment any possible deficiencies. Organic green foods and colorful fruits are the best source of antioxidants. You already know their importance in today's toxin-loaded environment.

> *Please eat organic – green foods grown conventionally can be loaded with high levels of pesticides.*

○ As emphasized earlier, taking vitamin C is crucial. You can hardly get enough of this immune boosting vitamin. Eat organic citrus fruits and berries and, by all means, take a multivitamin that contains 500 mg of vitamin C such as Ultimate Living Multi-Vitamin. The information we have provided should lead you to investigate the additional supplements needed by your immune system.

Eat a diet low in saturated fat. The American diet is saturated in fat. Drive down any commercial boulevard and what do you see? Fast foods and that generally refers to fried foods. Plus, foods high in fat are comforting, filling. We have to learn to become satisfied on foods rich in nutrients and fiber rather than saturated fat. A diet rich in organic fruits and vegetables is very important for a strong immune system. Excess fat hampers the ability of the body to fight off bacteria and free radicals. Lowering saturated fat, hydrogenated oils, and transfatty acids in the diet can be accomplished by limiting the intake of fried foods and making low fat and low calorie meal substitutions.

○ De-stress! A study published in The New England Journal of Medicine found that colds and flu are more likely to strike when a person is under psychological stress. Cancer researchers are definitely linking cancer to stress. Find time each day to relax. Take a warm bath, take a leisurely walk, keep a journal. Relax your mind and your body and, most importantly, learn to put things in their proper place–most things are really not worth worrying about.

○ Get eight hours of sleep or more a night. An exhausted body is open to infection and disease, not to mention you can never operate at peak performance if you are not rested. We believe that our bodies go through a detoxification and elimination process between the hours of 11 p.m. and 1 a.m. Therefore it is important to go to bed by 11 p.m.

○ Drink plenty of pure water daily. We recommend that you take your body weight and divide it by two. This will give you the amount of ounces of water you should consume each day. For instance, a woman who weighs 140 pounds needs about 70 ounces of water daily.

Since the thymus gland plays an important role in a healthy immune system, it requires some special attention, especially since it shrinks as we grow older and it can become lazy as well.

The thymus is located in the upper part of the chest behind the breastbone. It is a haven for the immune-system cells that help fight infection. You can energize the thymus by tapping on the middle of your breastbone for approximately five minutes each morning.

In Laurie Garrett's book *The Coming Plague*, she describes a world out of balance where we are doomed to be bombarded by infectious diseases. In reality, we already live in that world, and our most powerful defense is our own natural immune defense system.

We live in a crowded world. Movies, malls, airplanes are all places to catch infections passed between individuals. So what can we do?

○ *Remember to use antibiotics wisely. If your physician prescribes an antibiotic, take it as prescribed and take all of it.*

○ *Take a friendly bacteria supplement such as acidophilus. Remember that there are many environmental factors that disrupt your body's natural balance. The friendly bacteria that guard the intestines from infectious bacteria are often depleted by such factors as preservatives in food, chlorinated water, carbonated beverages, and stress. Much of the immune response in the body takes place in the intestinal tract so keeping it healthy and in balance is very important. Yogurt with live, active cultures is a good source of friendly bacteria.*

○ *Take a complete enzyme to aid in the digestive process. A complete enzyme contains amylase (breaks down carbohydrates, starches, and sugars), protease (breaks down protein), lipase (breaks down fat), and cellulose (breaks down fiber).*

○ *Do not use acid blockers or antacids. Stomach acid is crucial to both digestion and immunity. An enzyme supplement will help to eliminate digestive discomfort such as acid reflux, heartburn, indigestion, and IBS (irritable bowel syndrome). Most of the time, digestive discomforts are actually caused by incomplete absorption rather than too much acid.*

Chapter One: The Immune System

As mentioned earlier, sometimes our bodyguard turns against us. A key role of the immune system is its ability to differentiate between foreign invaders and the body's own cells. When it fails to make this distinction, the result is autoimmune disease. One of the most common autoimmune diseases is **rheumatoid arthritis**. This debilitating disease results from an immune reaction that attacks joint tissues, causing damage to the joints and eventually crippling the person afflicted.

Multiple sclerosis is one of the most debilitating autoimmune diseases. In this disease the immune system generates lymphocytes that attack and destroy nerves, ultimately leading to paralysis. Certain forms of **diabetes** are caused by an autoimmune reaction that destroys cells in the pancreas that produce insulin, the hormone required to control the levels of insulin in the blood.

Fibromyalgia, once thought of as a phantom disease, is now known to be one of the autoimmune responses and a form of arthritis. Often disabling, fibromyalgia causes widespread pain in the muscles, tissues, and joints. It also causes sleep disorders and great fatigue.

While autoimmunity is caused by inappropriate immune responses against self-antigens, the immune system can also go haywire against foreign antigens, a response known as hypersensitivity or allergies. **Allergies** are caused by an extreme immune response to a foreign antigen that would not ordinarily bother people. Some people become so sensitive that the response is dangerous as with those who are so allergic to nuts that eating them can trigger anaphylactic shock. **Asthma** is another common, disabling allergic reaction. While pollution itself does not seem to be the cause of asthma, it is certainly a trigger.

Boosting the immune system is one way of helping to diminish symptoms of autoimmune disorders as well as allergies.

Green Foods and the Immune System

The foundation of a healthy diet and, consequently, of a healthy immune system is a variety of foods that include plenty of organic green foods, grains, nuts, fruits, and vegetables. But our food sources have been so seriously compromised by depletive farming practices and other environmental factors that our fruits and vegetables lack many of the vital nutrients our forefathers enjoyed. It is, in fact, probable that the vitamins and minerals we need to enhance our immune systems are no longer present in many of our food sources.

Modern farm practices have increased our incidents of disease. Food animals are raised too quickly with the use of hormones, antibiotics, and steroids. Often products are processed into frozen foods that add even more chemicals and preservatives. It is likely that we are slowly being poisoned by our own diets. In addition, modern farm practices and over-farming have leeched vital nutrients from the soil, resulting in our food supply being depleted of much of the nutrition we need to keep our immune systems up and running at peak performance. "Eating right" has become more and more difficult.

While the new federal diet guidelines for fruit and vegetable consumption have increased from five servings to nine to thirteen servings per day (a serving is about half a cup), most of us don't even get close to the recommended amount. Most people in the U.S. eat only a few or no fruits and vegetables a day. With our immune systems being thus compromised, is it any wonder that disease and disability are on the rise?

It is urgent that we begin to take steps toward eating more beneficial foods. Dark green vegetables, for example, contain twenty times more essential nutrients than other foods. They are rich in antioxidants, vitamins, minerals, fiber, calcium, enzymes, protein, essential amino acids, and many other nutrients needed to cleanse, balance, detoxify, and regenerate our bodies. Green foods such as wheat grass, barley grass, spirulina, and green kamut help the body neutralize and reduce toxins while building the immune system.

Nutritional scientists and health experts agree that phytochemicals and phytonutrients found in green foods are essential for optimum health and the absorption of nutrients. Phytochemicals and phytonutrients are found naturally in all plant life, including fruits and vegetables, and they give plants their medicinal qualities. Consuming the proper amount of phytonutrients is very important to maintain good health and quality of life.

If we fail to eat green leafy vegetables on a daily basis, valuable cleansing, cell-building, and eliminative functions fail to work properly. This contributes to a compromised immune system and ultimately leads to degenerative disease.

In addition, green foods are rich in hundreds of active, natural enzymes. While we come into this world with enough enzymes to last us the rest of our lives, modern lifestyles and the environment are depleting our bodies' reserves. Enzymes are the chemical building blocks for our bodies and are essential for

> **Green foods are truly the superstars *of nutrition and, in fact, may hold the power to heal, nourish, and restore health! They help the body's ability to detoxify, fight those pesky free radicals, reduce inflammation, and assist in increasing oxygen carrying red blood cells.***

nutrient absorption. They help in proper digestion and in fighting off bacteria, carcinogens, and viruses. Enzymes also help bring our bodies into proper pH balance. If this balance is upset, cell metabolism suffers, which can lead to fatigue or, even worse, serious health problems.

Green foods also supply our body with a rich source of vegetable proteins. These proteins enhance the immune system, increase reproductive functions, and serve as building blocks for lean connective tissue. Strong connective tissues increase the strength of bone and muscular structure. This is very important for those at risk of osteoporosis. It is clear that to meet the needs of the body it is urgent that we eat green foods.

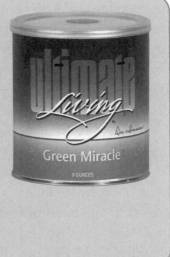

Ultimate Living Green Miracle, for example, a superior formulation, contains over 82 nutrients giving you over 8,000 milligrams of organic and all-natural ingredients. It is the cornerstone of our nutritional products. Three scoops per day is equal to a pound and a half of organic fruits and vegetables and provides the daily requirement of nutrients to keep the immune system healthy and strong. We call it "A Health Food Store in a Can."

In today's hectic society, however, it may frequently seem almost impossible to consume the required servings of fruits and vegetables, but it is not as difficult as it appears. A good green foods supplement is a great way to insure you are consuming your daily minimum requirement, and there are many green foods supplements on the market and some are quite good.

Let's Get Back to Basics

The time has indeed come for us to get back to basics. Think about it. Americans, as a culture, have complicated their lives. Isn't it more trouble to get in your car, go to the drive thru, and consume all things unhealthy than it would be to slice some cantaloupe and eat it with a half cup of cottage cheese on a bed of romaine lettuce? A healthy, low-calorie lunch might take five minutes to prepare, especially if you have thought about it in advance. By washing and bagging organic lettuce and greens every weekend, you will have them to use all week. You can do the same with fruits and veggies. You will have ready-made, inexpensive, healthy lunches all week. Add a cup of green tea with a slice of lemon and you have nourished your body and added valuable antioxidants.

Organic fruits and vegetables contain no harmful chemicals. Organic foods also contain higher amounts of minerals, vitamins, and essential nutrients. Plus, they are not treated with pesticides or preservatives so they do not strain the immune system. Organic fruits and veggies often are not as pretty as produce that has been sprayed, waxed, and preserved, but they do not create extra work for your immune system. Please eat organic whenever possible.

While fruits and vegetables should be the bulk of what you eat daily, a diet must be well-balanced to include all food categories. You need whole grains and protein as well as some fat everyday. In addition, water is essential to keep the body hydrated and flushed of harmful toxins. You should be drinking eight to ten glasses of pure water everyday.

Exercise regularly. Your activity does not have to be complicated. It can include a simple walk around the block, getting a massage, stretching, or taking the stairs instead of the elevator. If you do not move, your lymphatic system that drives your immune system will become blocked and toxins will remain in our body.

Once again, **REST**. Rest is the restorative process for your immune system. Rest your mind and your body.

Finally, supplement your diet with quality formulations. According to Congress, Public Law 103-417, 103rd Congress, 1994, scientific studies prove "that there is a link between ingestion of nutrients or dietary supplements and the prevention of chronic diseases such as cancer, heart disease, and osteoporosis, and clinical research has shown that several chronic diseases can be prevented simply with a healthful diet, such as a diet that is low in fat, saturated fat, cholesterol, and sodium, with a high proportion of plant-based foods."

Special Considerations for Flu Season

There is evidence that taking vitamin C may help prevent influenza. According to a study presented at the 60th Anniversary Meeting of the American Academy of Allergy, Asthma, and Immunology, people who take daily doses of vitamin C can boost their immune system, potentially protecting themselves from viruses and colds.

Drink plenty of water to keep your tissues hydrated. Healthy moist membranes are more likely to resist viruses.

Wash your hands before you prepare food and before you eat.

Fruits and vegetables contain vitamins, minerals, and natural substances that help keep you healthy. Flu season is not the time to neglect a healthy diet.

If you are healthy, you will be more resistant to the flu, or at least you may be able to recover faster.

Illness does not occur without cause. It occurs when our immune system has been compromised. Understanding the role that nutrients play in our health is vital in the fight against illness. Follow the advice provided in this chapter and you will be helping your immune system to remain your best defense against disease and your best asset in achieving optimum wellness.

An Amazing Immune System Booster

The Ojibwa Indians of Canada used an herbal formula consisting of four herbs to treat disease and illness. At the turn of the century, the wife of a Canadian gold miner developed breast tumors. An old Ojibwa medicine man told her about the herbal healing tea and offered to make it for her. Since her only other option was to have surgery, which could have been a death sentence during that time, she opted to try the herbal healing tea. The medicine man taught her which herbs to use and how to prepare them into a tea to drink twice a day. The documented story states that her breast tumors disappeared without surgery.

In 1922, the same lady met a nurse named Rene Caisse and told her the story and how to make the tea. The nurse found the opportunity to experiment with the tea. Her aunt and her mother were both terminal cancer patients. Both women completely recovered. Over the next fifty years, working with prominent physicians, Nurse Caisse used the herbal tea to successfully treat thousands of cancer patients. All benefited in many ways and lived much longer than anticipated.

Working with the famous doctor Charles Brusch, M.D., physician to the late President John F. Kennedy, Nurse Caisse changed and improved the formula. They struggled to create several formulas for different types of cancer. The main difference in the formulas was in the number of herbs. The different formulations could consist of five to eight different herbs. After extensive research, they found the formula that was superior and most effective.

In one instance, the natural healing herbal tea was used on a cancer patient who had diabetes and was insulin dependent. Nurse Caisse and the team of doctors with whom she was working were unsure how the tea would react with the insulin, so they took the patient off the insulin to administer the tea. Not only did the tumors vanish, but the diabetic condition disappeared as well.

History has shown and recorded the impact Nurse Caisse's formula made on total health and wellness. Scientists are still amazed at the herbal tea's healing properties and are continually researching reasons why this formula is so effective against many diseases.

Ultimate Living's own scientific team has discovered and utilized several new and exciting characteristics of this unique tea. Working with some of the top herbalists in the country, Ultimate Living's researchers have found this formulation may have a positive impact on many health-related issues. Some of the herbs in the formula are anti-parasitic; one acts as a natural painkiller; and another herb is known as the single best blood purifier. Ultimate Living is learning more everyday about the wonders of this gift from the Ojibwa Indians. We receive testimonials and reports daily about how **Immune Support Formula** has impacted health problems such as diabetes, arthritis, cataracts, polyps, tumors, parasites, and even high blood pressure. Although there is a long list of unrelated health concerns that seem to be affected by **Immune Support Formula**, the answer may be in the blood. The Ojibwa Indians say, "If you can clean the blood, the body can heal. But if you do not clean the blood, the body will never truly get well." Perhaps there is a great deal of truth in this statement. Ultimate Living's **Immune Support Formula** is made with the wisdom of ancient peoples coupled with the knowledge of modern science.

Ultimate Living Immune Support Formula

Helps to:

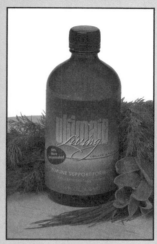

- *purify the blood*

- *improve pancreatic function*

- *regulate blood sugar levels*

- *stimulate and strengthen immune system function*

- *increase oxygen levels in the blood*

- *reduce pain*

- *detoxify the colon and liver*

- *eliminate parasites*

- *supply nutrients and vitamins*

Chapter Two

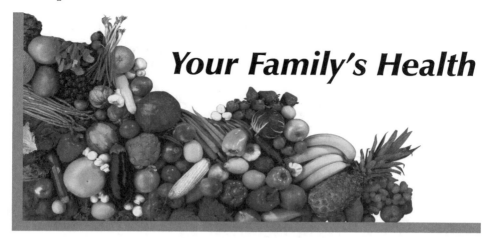

Your Family's Health

Sickness is of great concern to all families. Illness can cause financial woes, take an emotional toll, and disrupt a normal lifestyle. Keeping you and your family physically and spiritually healthy is paramount to a happy family life.

It is our responsibility as parents to pass on good practices to our children–habits that will endure. The best way to teach them a healthy lifestyle is to set a good example by eating nutritious foods, getting plenty of physical activity, and avoiding bad habits such as smoking and alcohol consumption. By practicing your faith, you will be setting an example for your children that will give them strength and encouragement throughout their lives.

Women have very specific health problems. Nutrition and lifestyle play a vital role in how well a woman can handle all of her daily activities and those of her family. As women age, there are many health considerations that must be addressed in order to have a healthy and productive middle-age.

In an effort to support families and to achieve success, men suffer from stress related illnesses. It is often up to the women in their lives to guide them toward taking care of their health.

Seniors have much to offer. They can be the pillar in a family and have experience and knowledge to share with loved ones and others. Seniors need to have good information to enable them to spend gratifying and productive lives.

Helpful Nutrition Notes

Food recommendations are almost always in servings. To clear up confusion on what actually constitutes a serving from the various food groups, use the following guide.

One food serving consists of:

Fruit	1 medium piece of fresh fruit
	1/2 cup chopped or canned fruit
	3/4 cup fruit juice
	1/4 cup dried fruit
Vegetables	3/4 cup vegetable juice
	1/2 cup other vegetables, cooked or raw
	1 cup raw, leafy vegetables
Whole Grains	1 slice of bread or a small roll
	1/2 bagel or English muffin
	1 oz. cold cereal
	1/2 cup cooked cereal, rice, or pasta
	3 or 4 small or 2 large crackers
Dairy	1 cup milk or yogurt
	1/2 cup of cottage cheese
	1 1/2 oz. of natural cheese (about the size of your thumb)
Proteins	2 to 3 oz. cooked lean meat, poultry, or fish
	1/2 cup cooked dried beans
	1 egg white
	2 tablespoons nut butter

Dietary Recommendations

The latest dietary recommendations for adults include:

▷ *9-13 servings of fruits and vegetables per day*

▷ *2-3 servings of protein per day*

▷ *2-3 servings of dairy per day for men*

▷ *3-4 servings of dairy per day for women*

▷ *2 servings of dairy per day for children older than toddlers*

▷ *4 servings of dairy per day for teens, pregnant women, and lactating mothers*

▷ *Limit your intake of fats–most of your fat intake should come from seeds and nuts as well as healthy oils such as olive, flax, or macadamia.*

Please remember:

● *Conventionally grown produce contains environmental toxins and pesticides.*

● *Conventionally produced dairy products and meats contain hormones and preservatives.*

● *Please buy organic whenever possible.*

Physical Activity

Our children are being exposed to less physical activity in school as physical education programs give way to computer classes. We, as parents, must instill the importance of consistent physical activity and exercise. Physical activity does not necessarily mean that you insist your son or daughter participate in sports. Hiking, bicycling, even gardening are all activities that you and your kids can enjoy together. Teaching your children an appreciation of nature encourages them to spend time outdoors rather than being glued to the computer or television.

Toys today are not designed to exercise children's bodies, only their hand-eye coordination. If you expose them to the wonders of the out of doors, they will be less inclined to bury themselves in the wonders of cyberspace.

Tips for raising healthy kids:

☆ *Don't buy junk food. Start your kids on fresh fruits, and the fruits will become their "sweets."*

☆ *Observe what your child buys for him or herself and discourage sodas and sugary wasted calories.*

☆ *Expose them to a variety of foods from infancy forward. It is easy to mash whatever vegetable you are serving. Remember children eat tiny portions. Don't overwhelm them. You will also be setting an example of proper portion size.*

★ *After age two, you should start your child on a good multivitamin that builds healthy bones, stimulates brain function (essential fatty acids), and helps prevent ADD/ ADHD.*

★ Ultimate Living Multi-Vitamin 4 Kids with Green Miracle is a terrific way to give your child a nutritional head start.

★ *Encourage your child to drink water or skim milk instead of sugar-loaded fruit drinks.*

★ *Discourage soda!*

★ *Make physical activity part of your daily routine with your family. A walk or a bike ride after dinner can be wonderful time together.*

★ *Do not allow your child to park in front of the television or video games.*

★ *Children should not have computers or televisions in their rooms. These items should be placed in a family area.*

Talk to Your Children

It is never too soon to talk to your children about the health hazards and dangers of tobacco, alcohol, and drug abuse.

Statistics show that the children of smokers are more apt to smoke and that the children of alcoholics are more likely to drink themselves. These are definitely examples of practicing what you preach.

Spending time with your kids is the best way to keep them out of trouble. The more time you spend with them, the more likely they will feel comfortable talking to you about their worries and concerns. You want to be their guide and their example.

Some ideas for fostering good connections with your children include the following:

- *Establish "together time." Make time in your day to sit down to just be with your children–reading a book, taking a walk, or just talking.*

- *Eat together often. Meals are a great time to talk about the day and to bond.*

- *Be a living, day-to-day example of your value system. Show the compassion, honesty, generosity, and integrity you want to see in your child.*

- *Don't react in a way that will cut off further discussion. Listen to what your child says, and respect his or her thoughts.*

● *Emphasize what your child does right. Restrain the urge to be critical. Positive reinforcement works.*

● *Let your children know how much you care even when they are at fault.*

● *Get involved in your child's school, your neighborhood, and your community. You are responsible for parenting your child.*

● *Be a guide for your children. Offer to help with homework, in social situations, and with concerns about the future. Be there for them–to listen to them and to hear their needs and concerns.*

● *Provide an environment for your children where a foundation of mutual respect is the basis of your relationship into their adult years. Let them know that they can always count on you.*

● *Be a spiritual example for your children.*

● *Teach your children to pray. It has been shown that prayer makes a difference during times of emotional and physical distress.*

There could not be a more difficult job than parenting these days. Just remember it is not our responsibility to be perfect parents or to raise perfect children. That effort would produce stress for both you and your children.

Rather, create a healthy, loving atmosphere where your child can develop and flourish into the person that he or she is meant to be.

Chapter Three

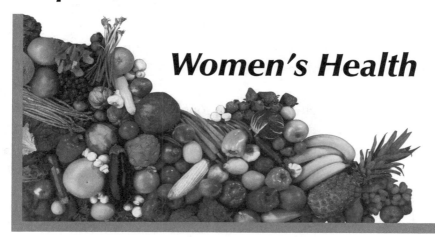

Women's Health

W omen have unique health issues and needs. Nutrition is a key factor from childhood through adolescence, pregnancy, menopause, and beyond. As nurturers, women often neglect themselves to look after their families and loved ones. In order to take better care of their families, women must take care of themselves.

A woman's specific health needs almost always relate to reproduction and the reproductive system. One of the best things a woman can do to protect her health is to make regular annual visits to her gynecologist. An annual Pap smear is recommended for all women beginning at the age of eighteen or whenever she becomes sexually active. The Pap smear is highly effective in detecting cervical cancer as well as pre-cancerous conditions. A base-line mammogram should be taken at age forty, and annual breast exams and mammograms should follow. Mothers should teach their daughters about breast self-examination at puberty so that the practice will have become a habit by the time they reach womanhood.

All adult women should have basic annual screenings that include height, weight, and blood pressure. At age fifty, all women should have a screening for colorectal cancer.

Staying fit and healthy throughout a woman's lifetime begins with eating a balanced diet, maintaining a proper weight, and making a lifelong practice of exercise. Establishing relationships and friendships is not only a good way to "stay young"; the caring and the support of others are proven to have positive effects on our health.

In addition, researchers have definitive proof that practicing your faith regularly and becoming a part of a spiritual community not only create feelings of security and belonging, but also affect your health and longevity positively.

Breast Cancer

Breast cancer is the most common cancer among women. Approximately 215,990 new cases of invasive breast cancer (Stages I-IV) are diagnosed annually. Another 59,390 women will be diagnosed with in situ cancers, non-invasive forms of the disease.

Risk Factors

Many factors can influence a woman's risk of getting breast cancer, but having one or more risk factors does not necessarily mean that a woman will get breast cancer. Some women with one or more breast cancer risk factors never develop the disease, while the majority of women with breast cancer have no apparent risk factors. Even when a woman has a risk factor, there is no way to prove that it was the actual cause of breast cancer. Risk factors for breast cancer include both those that cannot be changed, such as genetics and age, and those that can be changed, such as lifestyle.

These risk factors include:

Age

As a woman ages, her risk of breast cancer also increases. About seventy-seven percent of women with breast cancer are over age 50 at the time of diagnosis. Women between the ages of 20 and 29 account for only 0.3 percent of breast cancer cases.

Genetics

Changes (or mutations) of certain genes may cause some cells to become cancerous. Recent studies have shown that up to ten percent of breast cancer cases are hereditary.

Personal history

Women who have had breast cancer in one breast are three to four times more likely to develop breast cancer in the opposite breast than women who have never had breast cancer.

Previous breast biopsy showing benign conditions

Women who have previously had breast biopsies showing benign (non-cancerous) conditions may have a slightly higher risk of developing breast cancer. Women with fibrocystic change are not at increased risk for breast cancer (symptoms of fibrocystic breasts include lumpiness, tenderness, areas of thickening, cysts, or breast pain).

Menstrual periods

Women who begin menstruating at an early age (before age 12) and those who reach menopause after age 50 have an increased risk of breast cancer.

Women who breast feed have a lower incidence of breast cancer.

Alcohol

Most health care providers agree that daily alcohol consumption increases breast cancer risk. A recent study on alcohol and breast cancer revealed that women who consume two to five alcoholic beverages each day were found to have a slightly higher risk of developing invasive breast cancer compared to women who do not drink alcohol.

Smoking

Smoking increases a woman's chance of developing several types of cancer, including breast cancer.

Diet

There is a much higher incidence of breast cancer in areas with high fat diets (such as the United States) than in areas with low-fat diets (such as Japan). However, the link between diet and breast cancer risk is complicated and is affected by the type of fat in a woman's diet. Monounsaturated fats, such as canola oil or olive oil, have been linked to lower breast cancer risk, while a diet high in polyunsaturated fats, such as corn oils, tub margarine, and saturated fats in meats, is associated with a higher risk of breast cancer.

Weight

The link between weight and breast cancer risk is controversial. Several new studies suggest that overweight (obese) women who gained weight as adults are at an increased risk of developing breast cancer, but women who have been overweight since childhood are not at any significantly higher risk. Also, overweight women who take hormone replacement therapy may be at greater risk of developing breast cancer.

Previous radiation therapy

Women whose breast/chest area was exposed to radiation therapy during childhood are at higher risk of developing breast cancer, especially if radiation was used to treat Hodgkin's disease. In general, the younger the woman was when exposed to radiation, the greater the risk that she will develop breast cancer.

Hormone replacement therapy (HRT)

A woman's risk of breast cancer increases if she takes hormone replacement therapy (HRT). HRT is at the forefront of discussion in the medical community as never before. Hormone therapy is a treatment used to supplement the body with either estrogen alone or estrogen and progesterone. Large numbers of baby boomers are entering menopause every day. Simultaneously, doctors are realizing that HRT is not the answer to menopause they thought it was when they began to prescribe these dangerous drugs in the 1960s. At that time, unfortunately, not much was known about the drugs since little testing had been done. Pharmaceutical companies continued to push these drugs well into the 1980s because they claimed that they lowered women's risk of heart disease, stroke, and osteoporosis.

Independent researchers began testing these claims as well as studying more closely the side effects of long-term use of HRT. Their findings were astonishing! HRT drugs were actually increasing the risk of cancer by a shocking amount. When doctors finally launched a large-scale study involving thousands of women, they found that hormones increased a woman's risk of fibrocystic breasts, edema, uterine fibroids, and endometrial cancer and caused so many additional cases of breast cancer, stroke, blood clots, and heart attacks that the study was stopped years before it would have been completed. Five months after the study was halted, the federal government added estrogens to its list of known human carcinogens. These side effects are just the extremely dangerous ones. There are many recorded cases of migraine headaches, monthly bleeding, irregular spotting, decreased libido, dizziness, skin discoloration, and increased breast density and tenderness, to name a few. Neither list looks appealing when you actually weigh the pros and cons of taking HRT.

Breast Cancer Screening

Many women think that because breast cancer doesn't run in their families, they have nothing to worry about. Actually, ninety to ninety-five percent of the time, health professionals cannot determine why a woman gets breast cancer.

There are screening and examinations that can detect breast cancer early when it is very treatable.

To find breast cancer early, the National Cancer Institute recommends:

> *Women in their forties and older should have mammograms every one to two years.*

> *Women who are at higher than average risk of breast cancer should talk with their health care providers about whether to have mammograms before age forty and how often to have them.*

Many physicians and researchers also recommend:

- An annual clinical breast exam in which the health care provider examines the breasts while the woman is standing or sitting up and lying down. The woman may be asked to raise her arms over her head, let them hang by her sides, or press her hands against her hips. The health care provider looks for differences between the breasts, including unusual differences in size or shape. The skin of each breast is checked for a rash, dimpling, or other abnormal signs. The nipples may be squeezed to see if fluid is present.

● Monthly breast self-exams to check for any changes in the breasts. It is important to remember that breast self-exams cannot replace regular screening mammograms and clinical breast exams.

Dietary Guidelines for Breast Cancer

Women can reduce their risk for breast cancer and improve their overall health by following some specific dietary guidelines. Avoiding alcohol; eating fruits, vegetables, whole grains, and low-fat foods; and maintaining a healthy weight can all play a part in breast cancer prevention.

Limit Alcohol Consumption

Studies have shown a relationship between alcohol consumption and an increased risk for breast cancer. An average of more than two to five alcoholic drinks per day appears to increase the risk of breast cancer. This increased risk appears to be highest for post menopausal women. Women should know that enjoying an occasional drink a few days a week should not increase the risk for breast cancer. Women with a higher risk for breast cancer, however, should consider limiting or avoiding alcohol.

Soy

Soybeans and soy products such as tofu, tempeh, soymilk, and soy nuts contain compounds that can help lower elevated cholesterol and may play a "cancer protecting" role in the diet. While the protective effects of soy on breast cancer are far from proven, soy is a high protein, cholesterol free, and low saturated fat food. It may be worthwhile to include more soy foods in the diet as a meat replacement. Of note, it is not recommended that people take soy supplements (such as genistein or concentrated soy isoflavones in drink powders) until soy's role in breast cancer prevention is clearer.

Organic Fruits and Vegetables

Fruits, vegetables, and whole grains are known to keep the body healthy and less prone to diseases, possibly including breast cancer. These foods are also a great source of chemicals called antioxidants. Antioxidants repair damage that occurs naturally in our cells. A good mix of these types of foods contains much needed nutrients and vitamins.

> **Ultimate Living Green Miracle** *provides the perfect blend of organic fruits and vegetables to enhance the ability of the body's cells to fight disease.*

Fats

Some studies have shown that low-fat diets help prevent breast cancer. Other studies, however, are in disagreement regarding the role of fat in a woman's diet and the associated risk for breast cancer. Weight gain after menopause raises the risk of breast cancer, so a low-fat diet helps avoid weight gain and lowers the risk of cancer. Health experts agree that a low-fat diet has many known positive health benefits. A low-fat diet can significantly reduce a woman's risk for heart disease, obesity, and other health problems.

Even though the role of diet in breast cancer prevention has not been proven conclusively, by eating a well-balanced diet, a woman can feel confident that she is helping to ensure health and longevity. Before making any dietary changes or beginning a supplement program, you should always talk to your healthcare provider.

Heart Disease in Women

Heart disease has been largely ignored in women as a major health issue until recent years. It is now known that women may experience completely different symptoms of heart disease than do men. Since the initial research on heart attack and stroke were performed mainly on men, there was very little information specific to women on these illnesses.

On January 31, 2005, Reuters Health reported that even with new, more objective criteria, women are still less likely than men to have their heart condition accurately diagnosed as a heart attack. This area is currently under special scrutiny with many new treatments and guidelines tailored for women.

Statistics

The National Coalition of Women with Heart Disease provides the following startling statistics:

☆ Eight million American women are currently living with heart disease–ten percent of women ages 45-64 and twenty-five percent age 65 and over. Six million women today have a history of heart attack and/or angina or both.

☆ Thirteen percent of women age 45 and over have had a heart attack. 435,000 American women have heart attacks each year; 83,000 are under age 65, and 9,000 are under age 45. Their average age is 70.4.

☆ Four million women suffer from angina, and 47,000 of them were hospitalized in 1999.

☆ Forty-three percent of deaths in American women, or nearly 500,000, are caused by cardiovascular disease (heart disease and stroke) each year.

☆ 31,837 women die each year of congestive heart failure (62.6 percent of all heart-failure deaths).

☆ The age-adjusted rate of heart disease for African American women is seventy-two percent higher than for white women.

☆ African American women ages 55-64 are twice as likely as white women to have a heart attack, and thirty-five percent are more likely to suffer from coronary artery disease.

☆ Women who smoke risk having a heart attack nineteen years earlier than non-smoking women.

☆ Women with diabetes are two to three times more likely to have heart attacks.

☆ High blood pressure is more common in women taking oral contraceptives, especially obese women.

☆ Thirty-nine percent of white women, fifty-seven percent of Black women, fifty-seven percent of Hispanic women, and forty-nine percent of Asian/Pacific Islander women are sedentary and get no leisure-time physical activity.

☆ Twenty-three percent of white women, thirty-eight percent of Black women, and thirty-six percent of Mexican American women are obese.

☆ Thirty-eight percent of women and twenty-five percent of men will die within one year of a first recognized heart attack.

★ Thirty-five percent of women and eighteen percent of men who are heart attack survivors will have another heart attack within six years.

★ Forty-six percent of women and twenty-two percent of men who are heart attack survivors will be disabled with heart failure within six years.

★ Women are almost twice as likely as men to die after bypass surgery.

★ Women are less likely than men to receive beta-blockers, ACE inhibitors, or even aspirin after a heart attack.

★ More women than men die of heart disease each year, yet women receive only thirty-three percent of angioplasties, stents, and bypass surgeries; twenty-eight percent of implantable defibrillators; and thirty-six percent of open-heart surgeries.

★ Women comprise only twenty-five percent of participants in all heart-related research studies.

Coronary heart disease is the most common form of heart disease. Often referred to simply as "heart disease," it develops over time and can start as early as the teenage years. Heart disease does not go away–left untreated it will only worsen. Many times simply making lifestyle changes is all that is required to lessen the risk and onset of coronary heart disease. Studies have shown that women can lower their heart disease risk by as much as eighty-two percent simply by leading healthy lifestyles.

You are never too young to start improving your odds against heart disease. Most young women, however, frequently operate under the misconception that they are immune to heart disease and often have behavior and habits that will contribute to their risk.

For example,

- Most teen-age girls become less active than they were as children.

- Approximately fourteen percent of all American teenage girls are physically inactive.

- Over fifteen percent of girls between the ages of six and nineteen are overweight or obese.

- Thirty percent of all high school girls report using tobacco; eighty percent of all smokers begin before the age of eighteen.

During mid-life, a woman's risk for heart disease starts to rise dramatically. In part this is because a woman's body stops producing estrogen. Also, mid-life is a time when women tend to develop factors such as high blood pressure and elevated cholesterol levels that increase their risk for heart disease. One in fourteen women between the ages of 45 and 64 has heart disease.

Statistics related to this increase in risk for middle-age women include the following:

- At menopause, a woman's heart disease risk starts to increase significantly.

- Each year, about 88,000 women between the ages of 45-64 have a heart attack.

- About half of the women who have a heart attack before age 65 die within eight years.

> Heart disease rates are two to three times higher for postmenopausal women than for those of the same age who have not yet undergone menopause.

> Postmenopausal hormone therapy, with estrogen alone or with progestin–once thought to lower risk–is not recommended for long-term use to prevent heart disease. Consequently, it is now even more vital that women take other steps to reduce their heart disease risk.

> The lifetime risk of developing high blood pressure for women age 55 is about ninety percent. Beginning at age 45, more women than men have a total cholesterol reading of over 200 –borderline high or higher. About one in seven women over age 65 have coronary heart disease.

Statistics regarding older women and heart disease include the following:

- About twenty-four million women age 60 and older have high blood pressure.

- Most women over age 65 have obvious heart disease or "silent" atherosclerosis ("hardening of the arteries"). In silent atherosclerosis, there are no symptoms even though fatty plaques have built up in the arteries. Lowering cholesterol is especially important to keep heart disease and atherosclerosis from worsening.

- Each year, about 372,000 women age 65 and older have a heart attack.

- The average age for women to have a first heart attack is about 70, and women are more likely than men to die within a few weeks of a heart attack.

But it's never too late to take steps against heart disease. By taking action, older women, especially those who already have heart disease, can reduce their risk of developing heart-related problems.

> ***Because almost 6.7 million American women have heart disease, it is urgent that women be made more aware of the following:***
>
> ▷ Heart disease has no quick fix. Even if a special procedure, such as an angioplasty, is performed, heart disease will worsen unless treated with lifestyle changes and medication.
>
> ▷ About thirty-five percent of women who have had a heart attack will have another within six years.
>
> ▷ About half of the women who have a heart attack will be disabled with heart failure within six years. Heart failure is a life-threatening condition in which the heart cannot pump enough blood to supply the body's needs.

The American Heart Association has published specific guidelines for preventing and treating coronary artery disease in women. These guidelines address lifestyle changes, medications, supplements, and hormone therapy in menopausal women.

Lifestyle changes

- Stop smoking, and avoid secondhand smoke.
- Perform at least thirty minutes of moderate-intensity activity, such as brisk walking, at least five days a week.

● Eat a heart-healthy diet, and limit saturated fat to less than ten percent of calories and cholesterol intake to less than 300 mg; avoid trans fats.

● Keep your body mass index (BMI)* between 18.5 and 24.9 and your waist circumference less than 35 inches.

> ## ✳ Body Mass Index
>
> *Body mass index, or BMI, is a new term to most people. However, it is the measurement of choice for many physicians and researchers studying obesity. BMI uses a mathematical formula that takes into account both a person's height and weight. BMI equals a person's weight in kilograms divided by height in meters squared (BMI=kg/m2).*

● If you have coronary artery disease, be evaluated for depression.

● If you drink, do so in moderation (an average of one drink per day for women). If you do not drink, don't start.

● Reduce your salt intake to control hypertension.

Menopause

Women have many opportunities in the course of their lifetime to experience wonderful changes and transitions. Although many women find themselves struggling with unpleasant symptoms and emotional difficulties, menopause can be one of those opportunities.

Perimenopause, or pre-menopause, is a transitional stage of two to ten years prior to complete cessation of the menstrual period. Its average duration is six years and can appear in women from thirty-five to fifty years of age. This has not been a stage of women's lives much talked about, and a woman can find herself experiencing puzzling changes without knowing why. What is actually going on is a gradual decrease of estrogen.

As indicated below, the manifestations of perimenopause can vary.

☆ Menstrual cycles become shorter, longer, and/or irregular

☆ Flow becomes heavier or lighter

☆ Low blood sugar

☆ Fatigue several days before menstruation

☆ Weight gain

☆ Decreased sex drive

☆ Headaches–from mild migraines to those with aura and visual distortions

☆ Dry and/or itchy vulva, clitoris

☆ Increased incidence of yeast infections

The postmenopausal phase of a woman's life begins at menopause, which is one year after her last menstrual period. While postmenopause usually begins around age fifty, some women become postmenopausal in their mid 40s, while others do so in their later 50s. Postmenopause can begin early and suddenly after ovary removal or cancer treatment that damages the ovaries.

In early postmenopause, a woman's estrogen stabilizes at a low level. Although low estrogen helps reduce the risk of various types of cancer, it also leads to an increasing loss in bone density, sometimes resulting in osteoporosis. A variety of hormonal and nonhormonal treatments are available for postmenopausal women with perimenopausal symptoms and/ or long-term osteoporosis concerns. Women are generally encouraged to try nonhormonal treatment to avoid the cancer, heart, and dementia risks of hormone replacement therapy (HRT).

Hormone Replacement Therapy (HRT)

In 2002, a decision was made to stop one component of the Women's Health Initiative. At that point, researchers found that HRT did not live up to any of the supposed benefits but instead caused problems, some very serious, such as cancer. Scientists weighed both the risks and benefits of the combined therapy of estrogen plus progestin and concluded it could cause more harm than good by raising the risk of heart attack, strokes, and breast cancer. Then in July 2003, another analysis of data from the Women's Health Initiative study found that instead of sharpening the mind, hormones might double the risk of Alzheimer's and other forms of dementia.

Now we are told in the Journal of the American Medical Association (JAMA) that HRT is definitely responsible for an increase in breast cancer and, to make matters worse, that breast cancers associated with hormone replacement therapy are harder to diagnose, resistant to treatment, and more likely to be fatal.

For decades women have been relieving the unbearable symptoms of premenstrual syndrome (PMS) and menopause with synthetic hormones. HRT has long been regarded as a way to avoid that image of menopause that depicts women as sleep-deprived, over-weight, indecisive, exhausted, anxious, basically in a state of dysfunction for years while their families try to stay out of their way. Now women who are entering menopause are faced with a dilemma, and women who have been taking HRT through menopause and have decided to quit will be faced with recurring symptoms. What are they to do? Do they have to face that image again?

The answer is a resounding "NO!" There is another and a better way to eliminate hot flashes, night sweats, anxiety, and the whole laundry list of symptoms you may be experiencing.

Menopausal women may experience symptoms such as hot flashes, night sweats, mood swings, weight gain, sleeplessness, headaches, fatigue, vaginal discomfort or infections, and bladder infections. Some women complain of irritability, tearfulness, and an inability to concentrate. Even though the vast majority of women in menopause experience some of these symptoms, they do not have to rule their lives. Now, in fact, many of the same doctors who prescribed HRT are suggesting natural products for their patients to help them gain relief from menopausal symptoms. Progesterone creams are at the top of the list of possible remedies as well as compounds containing phytoestrogens (plant-based estrogen).

Ultimate Living Harmony Cream contains a carefully chosen blend of natural progesterone, herbs, and phytochemicals that will help relieve many of the unpleasant symptoms of menopause.

Symptoms and Relief

A hot flash is a sudden sensation of intense body heat, often with profuse sweating and reddening of the head, neck, and chest. These symptoms can be accompanied by mild to severe heart palpitations, anxiety, irritability, and, rarely, panic. Hot flashes are a hallmark symptom of a woman's estrogen fluctuation around the time of her last menstrual period.

The actual cause of hot flashes is not well understood. Hot flashes are more common at night (night sweats) than during the day and are the main cause of sleep disruption for perimenopausal and postmenopausal women.

While some women will never experience hot flashes, others begin having them in their thirties. Hot flashes are most frequent and intense during the first two years of menopause when estrogen levels have dropped below a certain point. Sleep patterns usually improve within six to twelve months after hot flashes begin.

Tips for managing hot flashes:

➤ *Dress in layers so you can remove clothes as needed.*

➤ *Wear natural fabrics such as cotton and silk.*

➤ *Keep the room temperature cool or use a fan. You're more likely to have a hot flash in a warm environment than in a cool one.*

➤ *Sleep with fewer blankets.*

➤ *Drink cold beverages rather than hot ones.*

➤ *Limit your intake of caffeine and alcohol.*

➤ *Eat smaller, more frequent meals.*

➤ *Do not smoke.*

➤ *Use relaxation techniques such as yoga and biofeedback.*

➤ *Get regular physical exercise.*

➤ *Include plenty of low-fat, high-fiber foods in your diet.*

➤ *Use an all-natural progesterone cream.*

We now know that the chemicals in most deodorants are unhealthy. In fact, certain chemicals used to inhibit perspiration are downright dangerous. We recommend that you use an all natural deodorant that contains no aluminum or propylene glycol. These have both been linked to cancer.

> **Ultimate Living Natural Deodorant** *is an exclusive blend of natural ingredients essential for healthy underarm protection. Our Natural Deodorant encourages healthy blood circulation and does not contain propylene glycol or aluminum.*

Our culture has made it very unpopular to perspire. Remember the old commercial *Never let 'em see you sweat*. In reality, perspiring is one way the body eliminates toxins and waste. It is best to let your body do what is intended. Never use an antiperspirant.

There are ways to minimize the unpleasantness of PMS and menopause without jeopardizing your health by taking hormone replacement therapy. Remember that there is no better way to improve wellness than by eating right. Your diet should include plenty of dark green leafy veggies (great cancer preventatives) and fresh fruits. Experts now call for at least nine to thirteen servings of fruits and vegetables a day.

Try your best to cut back on fatty foods. They do more harm than good. Substitute steamed or grilled whenever possible. Invest in some good cookbooks and learn the art of seasoning to satisfy. And while a great piece of Belgian chocolate can't be beat, eat less sugar and fewer sweets. Menopause makes weight loss more difficult than ever, and sugar provides nothing but empty calories.

Pure drinking water helps to hydrate the body and to keep cells young. Make sure you are drinking pure water, not tap water loaded with chemicals. The best water is water that has been through a reverse osmosis process.

Carry a bottle of water with you and sip on it consistently. Thirst is the body's way of saying that it is becoming dehydrated, and dehydration is hard on your internal organs as well as your largest external organ, the skin. Take the time to go to your grocery or health food store and experiment with good bottled water. Buy several and have a tasting. Settle on the one you like best and drink it often. You should see a marked difference in your skin and know that you are helping to flush out toxins at the same time. Eight to ten eight-ounce glasses of water a day are recommended.

Don't forget your vitamins and minerals. Studies have shown that persons who take even a multi-vitamin daily can stave off disease and stay healthier than those who do not. If your diet is not all that it should be, then it is imperative that you take dietary supplements. Nothing can improve on good, wholesome food, but supplements can bridge the gap left by busy schedules.

Ultimate Living Multi-Vitamin provides all the nutrients your body needs plus it contains 400 IU of natural vitamin E.

Most people do not realize that much of our food supply is bereft of nutrition due to poor soil conditions, food storage, and transport as well as over-processing. Unless you can take the time, effort, and money to buy fresh organic fruits and vegetables, you are not receiving the total benefits that our food should supply. Poor nutrition can cause imbalances, including hormone imbalance!

Regular exercise has been proven to help relieve menopausal symptoms and stress! If you have not been exercising at all, then it is imperative that you start out slowly, for example, a thirty minute stroll in the morning or after dinner. You can build up to a steady pace, but any activity is better than none. Even something that seems passive, such as gardening, is good for you. And face it, activity that you are enjoying has another benefit;

it helps get rid of stress. You can't be worried and fretful while you are swimming or bicycling. So for at least thirty minutes a day, get up and move!

The real culprit of menopause is a lack of sleep and good rest. Menopause has such a bad name primarily because we become exhausted, and who can function at their best when they are tired? When sleeplessness occurs night after night, we really cannot cope. So make sure that, starting today, you take time to rest and relax, and tonight get in bed a little earlier. Be sure to adjust your bedroom to accommodate your body temperature; keep the room as cool as possible. Try sleeping in lightweight cotton night clothes, and do keep a big glass of pure water right beside the bed.

Natural Remedies

Phytoestrogens are a group of chemicals found in plants that can act like estrogen. Estrogen derived from plant sources or phytoestrogens can also help to regulate hormones.

More than 300 foods have been shown to contain phytoestrogens. Most food phytoestrogens are from one of three chemical classes, the isoflavonoids, the lignans, or the coumestans. Isoflavonoid phytoestrogens are found in beans from the legume family; soybeans and soy products are the major dietary source of this type of phytoestrogens. The fact that Asian women eat a diet high in soy proteins is another reason they are said to experience fewer menopausal complaints.

Lignan phytoestrogens are found in high fiber foods such as cereal brans and beans; flaxseeds contain large amounts of lignans. The coumestan phytoestrogens are found in various beans such as split peas, pinto beans, and lima beans; alfalfa and clover sprouts are the foods with the highest amounts of coumestans.

Women diagnosed with breast cancer should speak to their physicians and oncologists before taking certain supplements or consuming large amounts of foods that contain phytoestrogens.

Progesterone cream is one way to overcome the estrogen dominance syndrome that occurs at perimenopause and during menopause. Most menopausal symptoms are actually caused by an imbalance between a woman's estrogen and progesterone levels (estrogen levels exceed progesterone). By raising the progesterone levels with an effective, natural progesterone cream, many symptoms will abate. Wild yam, an excellent source of natural progesterone, is commonly the main ingredient in these creams along with other extracts such as burdock root, ginseng, black cohosh, calendula–all known to help relieve the menopause and PMS symptoms of hot flashes, night sweats, headaches, and water retention.

Black cohosh, milk thistle seed, red clover, hops, and flax are some specific supplements that will help to eliminate symptoms and increase energy levels during menopause.

➢ **Black cohosh** is an herb known for its estrogen-like effects. It aids in eliminating premenstrual symptoms, prevents menstrual cramps, and lightens the menstrual flow. It is effective in relieving hot flashes, night sweats, and PMS.

➢ **Red clover** is an herb containing phytoestrogens that assist in restoring hormone balance. It has properties similar to soy isoflavones and acts as a natural sedative for nervous exhaustion.

➢ **Hops** contains a form of estrogen that has the ability to relax and soothe. It is beneficial for relieving nervousness, pain, stress, insomnia, and muscle cramps.

➢ **Milk thistle** is thought to help ease headaches that often accompany PMS and menopause. It enhances liver function by inhibiting free radicals.

> ▷ **Flaxseed** has a significant impact on reducing the symptoms of menopause. Flax contains high levels of phytoestrogens effective in reducing hot flashes and other symptoms.

If you are over forty, you should consider taking two **Ultimate Living Hormone Balance** *capsules each day.*

Dong Quai is a natural herb that has been taken by Asian women for hundreds of years. Asian women have very few complaints of menopausal discomfort compared to Western women. Dong Quai is like a female ginseng, considered an overall sexual tonic, and is said to regulate the hormonal and menstrual cycle, relieving the complaints of perimenopause. This herb can make your menstrual flow heavier, so it is best to abstain from it during the week of your period.

It seems that water retention is a part of being female. It comes with menstruation and again with menopause. Foods that relieve water retention include (in order of effectiveness) asparagus, nettles, grapes, cucumbers, watermelon, parsley, celery, black tea, and green tea.

Calcium

While a proper balance of all minerals is important in maintaining optimum health, calcium takes on special importance during the menopausal years. To insure a positive calcium balance, avoid arthritis, prevent kidney stones, and create dense, flexible bones, we should all consume large amounts of calcium during the premenstrual years (please, tell your daughters and granddaughters). But for those of us who did not, it is never too late to start. Try to include an ample amount of calcium-rich foods in your daily diet and take a quality calcium supplement.

Ultimate Living Cal-Mag Plus *contains hydroxyapatite calcium, the most effective and absorbable form of calcium.*

Calcium-rich foods include:

Milk products	**Yogurt**
Cheese	**Greens**
Broccoli	**Sardines with bones**
Tofu	**Almonds**

Attitude

Women and men need to change their attitude about menopause. Menopause is meant to be a beautiful and natural change of life instead of the curse that it is so often thought to be. With the beginning of menopause, women are entering the golden age of their lives. They finally have reached a pinnacle of wisdom that comes only with age in years; and they are able to reflect clearly on love, spirituality, and the meaning of life with a knowing attitude and an ease such as they have never before experienced. At this age, women have finally settled into their skin. They know who they are because they have defined their individuality and have accepted themselves with all of their positive qualities as well as their shortcomings.

Remember, menopause is not a disease and cannot be prevented. It can, however, be managed! So starting today, take charge of menopause. Don't let it get the best of you. If you follow the simple changes discussed in this chapter, you will see a marked improvement in your overall well-being almost immediately.

Ultimate Living Hormone Balance combined with *Harmony Cream* will help your body slowly reduce your hormone levels over a longer period of time instead of all at once. The herbs we have so carefully selected to combine with our all-natural progesterone cream support your body with nutritious phytochemicals, acting as hormone precursors that your body needs and utilizes to manufacture hormones. Using our *Complete Hormone Program* correctly and following a healthy diet and lifestyle should alleviate the need for HRT; help restore mental clarity; reduce water retention; protect against heart disease, osteoporosis, and arthritis; increase protection against cancer; and enhance sleep. Most importantly, these products will reduce hot flashes and night sweats, the most common complaint of menopausal women. Finally, these products might actually restore peace in your home, in your workplace, and in your relationships.

Osteoporosis

Osteoporosis is often confused with osteoarthritis, the most common form of arthritis. In osteoporosis, the bones are thinning, and the term itself literally means thinning of bone. Osteoarthritis, on the other hand, is a wearing down of the cartilage protecting the bone. Osteoporosis is a condition where bone itself breaks down. Bones then become thin, brittle, and easily broken. For example, sneezing can cause an affected person's rib to break, or stumbling can lead to the fracture of one of the bones in the spine. The bones most commonly affected by osteoporosis are those in the hip, wrist, and particularly those in the mid-back. Osteoporosis usually appears in people after age forty, and women develop this disease four times more often than men.

There are many factors involved in causing osteoporosis. Bone is a living tissue that is continually growing and being removed. Bones usually reach their maximum mass when people are in their mid-thirties. At about age forty, bone begins to diminish (about one percent per year) so the bones start to become brittle.

Bone loss in women accelerates after menopause. Estrogen is a hormone that is important to maintaining bone strength; and once a woman enters menopause, her estrogen levels fall. This affects how her bones process calcium and may lead to a more rapid loss of bone. In men, low levels of the hormone testosterone may have the same effect.

A person's body type can also be a factor. Having a small frame and bone structure may increase the chances of getting osteoporosis.

Illnesses such as diabetes and rheumatoid arthritis may also cause bone loss. Eating disorders such as anorexia nervosa or bulimia can affect a person's estrogen level, therefore contributing to bone loss and the onset of osteoporosis. In addition, some medications, when taken in high doses, can diminish the body's ability to absorb calcium. These include cortisone/corticosteroids, anticoagulants, thyroid supplements, and some anti-convulsive drugs.

Because bone is a living tissue, it needs exercise to stay strong. If you are not active, your bones will become weaker over time. If you do not engage in regular activity and exercise throughout your life, you could increase your risk of developing osteoporosis. Bones also need nourishment from calcium, vitamin D, and phosphorous. A diet lacking foods that contain these vitamins and minerals contributes to bone loss. Foods rich in calcium are especially necessary in order to maintain healthy bones.

Preventing osteoporosis is much easier than curing it. If a person builds strong bones when young, bones will be able to withstand changes that can occur as we age. Parents need to instill good bone building habits in their children since the critical ages for bone development are between ten and thirty.

There are ways to combat osteoporosis and to ease symptoms as we age.

- Eat a well-balanced diet that includes foods rich in calcium (milk, cheese, yogurt, salmon, sardines, almonds, dark green leafy vegetables, and broccoli).

- Exercise regularly. Exercise helps rebuild bone and strengthens muscles. Walking, low-impact aerobics, and stationary cycling are all good forms of exercise. Swimming or other water exercises are good if you have too much pain and stiffness for other activities. In addition to preventing bone loss or rebuilding bone, exercise can also strengthen muscles. Having strong muscles increases flexibility. Weight bearing exercises are the most effective way to prevent or arrest bone loss. Weight bearing exercises do not necessarily have to include the use of weight. Even raking leaves, digging holes, or pushing a lawn mower can be considered weight-bearing exercise. The National Osteoporosis Foundation has listed the following as good weight-bearing exercises: walking, vigorous gardening/ yard work, jogging, impact aerobics, climbing stairs, cross-country skiing, soccer, tennis, dancing, inline skating, and hiking.

- Take it easy. Use your back, arms, and legs in safe ways to avoid putting stress on joints. Don't lug heavy grocery sacks–use a cart. Install handles in your bath or shower. Remember that osteoporosis means thinning bones, so breaks are a possibility, especially if you should fall.

- If you are overweight, start a weight loss program. Excess weight puts stress on your bones and joints.

- Excessive use of alcohol or caffeine-containing products such as tea, coffee, or some sodas can stop your body from absorbing calcium. Smoking also contributes to bone loss.

Ultimate Living Cal-Mag Plus contains hydroxyapatite calcium, the most absorbable form of calcium, which is ten times more effective than other types of calcium and assists in the prevention of bone loss. It also contains boron and vitamin D for maximum calcium retention. It is very important that calcium and magnesium be in the correct ratio. This means the dosage of magnesium should be exactly half that of calcium. For example, for every 1000 mg of calcium you would need 500 mg of magnesium for maximum benefit.

Anemia

Anemia is a condition in which your blood does not have enough hemoglobin. Hemoglobin is the protein in red blood cells that transports oxygen from your lungs to the rest of your body. Sometimes a lack of iron is the cause for anemia since the body requires iron to produce hemoglobin.

If you are anemic, you might experience paleness, fatigue, shortness of breath, or rapid heartbeat although often there are no symptoms.

If you suspect that you may be anemic, tell your physician. A simple blood test can detect anemia. There are many factors that can cause anemia, but the most common are

> **Lack of iron in the diet.** This is mostly a problem for children and young women. Children who drink a lot of milk and don't eat iron-rich foods and young women who follow "fad" diets may be at risk for iron deficiency.

▷ **Growth spurts.** Children occasionally become anemic during periods of rapid growth.

▷ **Pregnancy.** Women who are pregnant or who are breast feeding need 2½ times as much iron as men. Iron is often a suggested supplement for pregnant and lactating mothers.

▷ **Loss of Blood.** Heavy periods can cause anemia. Other factors could be bleeding from an ulcer or some other bleeding in the intestinal tract.

Some types of anemia are preventable by eating certain iron-rich foods.

These foods include:

Seafood

Dried fruits such as apricots

Prunes and raisins

Nuts

Beans, especially lima beans

Green leafy vegetables such as spinach and broccoli

Blackstrap molasses

Whole grain, iron-fortified breads and cereals (check the label)

B vitamins will prevent anemia. **Ultimate Living B Complex– Lingual** *is a complete B vitamin including B-12, B-6, and folic acid.*

Pregnancy

Many women wait until they suspect they might be pregnant before visiting the doctor–before taking health precautions at all.

Conception usually occurs about two weeks prior to a menstrual period. That means that by the time you think you may be pregnant, you have been so for several weeks; and during that time, your baby has developed facial features and organs, including the heart and the kidneys. Anything you have been eating or drinking can affect your baby. This is especially true if you smoke or are exposed to toxins. This is why it is important for you to prepare to become pregnant.

Remember that what you ingest your baby also ingests. If you consume colas and junk food, this will be the "nourishment" your baby receives. Pregnancy is a time when you need to be particularly mindful of your diet and nutrition. It is important that you speak with your physician before taking supplements, especially those containing herbs as there are some that are considered harmful to a developing fetus.

Folic acid deficiency has been linked to having babies with serious brain and spinal cord problems. You should take 500 mg of folic acid before becoming pregnant and 800 mg during pregnancy. Folic Acid can decrease the risk for neural tube defects (NTD's), which are birth defects of the baby's brain (anencephaly) or spine (spina bifida). NTD's happen when the spinal cord fails to close properly. Brain and spinal cord problems develop very early (about a month into the pregnancy).

*The combination of **Ultimate Living Multi-Vitamin** and **B Complex– Lingual** is an excellent way to sustain a healthy pregnancy.*

Physical Activity

The amount and the level of physical activity you do during your pregnancy are related to how fit you are when you become pregnant. Generally the more active you can be during your pregnancy, the easier your delivery will be. Walking is always a good option, but you need to discuss your exercise and physical activity with your physician.

Friendship

Women, it seems, find great pleasure in talking with their friends. Men, on the other hand, are more "doers" than talkers. They enjoy each other's company through activities such as fishing, golfing, and hunting.

And while women tend to "share" things and men tend to "do" things together, nonetheless, both men and women gain the same thing from friendships: longer, healthier lives.

"Friendship has a profound effect on your physical well-being," says Eugene Kennedy, Ph.D., professor of psychology at Loyola University of Chicago. As Professor Kennedy states, "Having good relationships improves health and lifts depression. You don't necessarily need drugs or medical treatment to accomplish this–just friends!"

And maybe one of the greatest health benefits of friendship is the youthfulness of extended life–of extra years of pleasure and satisfaction. Sharing special moments with our family and friends is irreplaceable in terms of the benefits to our health.

One of the first studies linking relationships and longevity was conducted by researchers in Alameda, California. They found that over a nine year period, people with the strongest social and community ties were the least likely to die young. Not surprisingly, more isolated people had the highest death rate. More recent studies confirm these findings. Redford B. Williams, M.D., director of the Behavioral Medicine Research Center and professor of psychiatry at Duke University Medical Center in Durham, North Carolina, sees a definite connection between friendship and longevity. His team studied 1,368 heart disease patients for nine years. "What we found," says Dr. Williams, "was that those patients with neither a spouse nor a friend were three times more likely to die than those involved in a caring relationship."

Michael Cunningham, Ph.D., professor of psychology at the University of Louisville in Kentucky says, "Women are much more likely to approach someone when they feel the need to meet someone new or just to talk. It's a healthy quality."

So-called "girl talk" isn't just fun. It's healthy!

Chapter Four

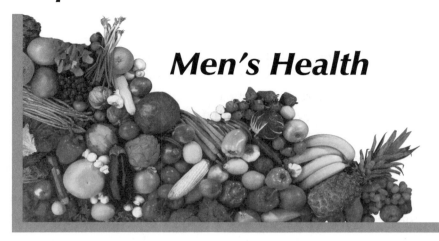

Men's Health

Men have special health concerns, but the good news is that many of the major health risks that men face can be prevented and treated if they are diagnosed early.

Benign Prostatic Hyperplasia (BPH)

The prostate is a walnut-sized gland located just below the bladder. Proper functioning of the prostate is important to bladder control as well as for normal sexual function.

While harmless, benign prostatic hyperplasia (BPH) is a common condition that can interfere with the urine's exit from the bladder, causing frequent urination, nighttime awakenings, and other uncomfortable urinary symptoms. While the exact cause of BPH is not known, more than half of the men over age 60 are afflicted. It often causes great discomfort.

Don't try to self-diagnose BPH. Although often benign, prostate problems should always be examined by a doctor to rule out other, more serious conditions, including prostate cancer. Consult a doctor if you develop symptoms of prostate problems (trouble urinating despite the urge, more frequent need to urinate, urinary leaking) or if you detect blood in your urine.

Saw Palmetto

Saw palmetto, also known as Serenoa repens or Sabal serrulatum, is an herb. The medicinal properties of saw palmetto are taken from the partially dried ripe fruit of the American dwarf palm tree indigenous to the coastal regions of the southern United States from the Carolinas and Florida to California. Taken from the olive-sized berries of the saw palmetto tree, saw palmetto acts as a remedy for benign enlargement of the prostate gland. Saw palmetto relieves the major symptoms of BPH. Numerous studies have shown that this herb reduces the number of times a sufferer feels the urge to urinate (including at night, thus reducing the number of nighttime awakenings), increases maximum urine flow, and minimizes the sensation that the bladder has not emptied. Painful urination may lessen as well. A recent analysis of several small clinical trials of saw palmetto published in The Journal of the American Medical Association (JAMA) found that men given saw palmetto were twice as likely to report a lessening of symptoms than those given a placebo.

Don't stop taking a prescription medication and start taking saw palmetto for prostate problems without discussing the change with your doctor. Despite some claims to the contrary, saw palmetto won't increase sexual vigor or increase your sperm count. Little is known about how high doses might affect your health. We recommend taking 320 mg daily; the amount that is in our **Men's Formula**.

Because the herb appears to affect hormone levels, men with prostate cancer or breast cancer, or anyone with a hormone-dependent illness, should first discuss the idea of taking saw palmetto with a doctor.

Also, since saw palmetto can affect prostate specific antigen (PSA) levels, be sure to let your doctor know that you are taking it before you undergo the test used to rule out prostate cancer.

Prostate Cancer

Because the incidence of prostate cancer is very common, prostate health is especially important. Prostate cancer is, in fact, the most common cancer among American men and the second leading cause of cancer death for men after lung cancer. The risk of prostate cancer increases with age. More than eighty percent of all prostate cancers are diagnosed in men over the age of sixty-five. In some men, prostate cancer is a slow-growing disease, and they will more than likely die of other causes rather than from prostate cancer. For others, the disease can be quite aggressive and require immediate treatment.

Symptoms of prostate cancer include:

- frequent urination or an inability to urinate

- trouble starting or holding back urine

- frequent pain or stiffness in the lower back, hips, or upper thigh

These same symptoms can be seen in a common non-cancerous condition, that of enlarged prostate. It is important that a man with these symptoms seek a professional diagnosis and treatment.

There are several tests for prostate cancer. A digital rectal exam can reveal tumors when the doctor feels the prostate to check for abnormalities. A blood test to detect the amount of prostate specific antigen (PSA) circulating in the bloodstream is another important method of diagnosing prostate cancer. If either the digital exam or the test for PSA is abnormal, the doctor may advise a biopsy, which involves inserting needles into the prostate to extract cells.

The treatment of prostate cancer is hotly debated. The side effects from treatment can have major impacts on a man's day-to-day life, impacts such as impotence and incontinence.

Faced with a number of possible treatment choices, it is vital that a man diagnosed with prostate cancer follow these guidelines before making any decisions:

- Gather as much information as possible about your specific condition, choices of treatment, and their possible side effects.

- Consider the side effects of each treatment choice and how they might affect both your physical and psychological well being.

- Seek out support groups and men who have gone through treatment. They can offer advice based on experience.

- Continue to watch for new information on your condition. Great strides are made everyday in the treatment of cancer.

Risk Factors

Risk factors for prostate cancer include the following:

> **Age:** There is a strong correlation between increasing age and developing prostate cancer. The incidence of prostate cancer increases steadily from fewer than one in 100,000 for men age 40 years to 1146 per 100,000 in men age 85 years. The median age at diagnosis of prostate cancer is 70.5. More than eighty percent of prostate cancers are diagnosed in men older than 65. Autopsy records indicate that seventy percent of men older than 90 have at least one region of cancer in their prostate.

➤ **Race:** African American men are 1.5-2 times more likely than white men to develop prostate cancer. African American men also appear to develop prostate cancer at an earlier age than white males.

➤ **Genetic factors:** Men who have a history of prostate cancer in their family, especially if it was a first-degree relative such as a father or brother, are at an increased risk. This risk may be two to three times greater than the risk for men without a family history of the disease.

➤ **Diet:** A diet high in fat has been associated with an increased risk.

➤ **Chemical agents:** Exposure to chemicals has been implicated in the development of prostate cancer.

While environmental factors seem to influence the development and progression of prostate cancer, the strongest environmental influence appears to be diet, specifically fat.

Fat consumption has been conclusively linked both to the development of prostate cancer and the death rate from this disease. The U.S. and western European countries have the highest death rates from prostate cancer and also the highest per capita fat consumption. In contrast, the Pacific Rim countries with the lowest death rates from prostate cancer also have the lowest fat consumption.

In Japan, an increase in prostate cancer risk was seen to be commensurate with the introduction of western-style diets and higher fat intake. It has been noted that men with a high fat consumption not only were more likely to develop prostate cancer, but they also developed a more aggressive form of the disease. It was reported that men with the highest intake of red meat had a risk of developing prostate cancer 2 ½ times greater than that of men with the lowest intake of red meat.

In 1981, an American Cancer Society survey of 750,000 individuals demonstrated a correlation between obesity and clinical prostate cancer.

Prostate Cancer Screening

Despite the prevalence of prostate cancer, many men are still uncomfortable discussing the topic. In fact, less than ten percent of men in the United States are screened for prostate cancer. So it is a disease that has many unanswered questions.

Early detection of prostate cancer is critical to successful treatment. Most prostatic cancers are initially detected through an elevated prostate specific antigen (PSA) test and a digital rectal exam (DRE). A DRE is a gloved-finger examination of the prostate through the rectum. The PSA test is a blood test used to help screen for prostate cancer. The only conclusive form of detection is biopsy. This is usually done with the aid of ultrasound.

To detect prostate cancer early, the American Cancer Society advises that all men over 50 have an annual prostate DRE and a PSA blood test. Many doctors, however, recommend that those at high-risk (African-American men and those men with a family history of prostate cancer) should begin testing as early as age 40.

The PSA blood test is used to check the enzyme normally produced by the prostate cells. PSA is not found in large amounts anywhere else in the body. A small amount of PSA normally leaks into the blood stream and can be detected with a simple blood test.

Higher levels of PSA can be associated with inflammation, enlargement, or prostate cancer. In other words, a mild to moderate increase in PSA does not always mean cancer. Often a higher PSA level can show that the prostate cancer is in its later stages and may have spread. Together, the PSA blood test and the DRE are used as tools to detect cancer early.

An abnormal PSA test result is defined as 4.0 ng/ml or higher. An elevated level does not necessarily mean cancer. The age of the patient, prostate size, or an infection may also have an influence on this level. Also, a patient may have a normal PSA level but still have prostate cancer. That is why it is imperative to have both a PSA test and a DRE.

Nutrition and Prostate Cancer

Dietary guidelines for the prevention of prostate cancer include the following:

- Limit the percentage of dietary fat to fifteen to twenty percent of total energy intake.

- Eat more than five servings of fruits and vegetables daily.

- Consume 25-35 g of dietary fiber daily.

- Consume 40 g of soy protein per day.

- Balance caloric intake with energy output.

- Consume 10 servings of lycopene rich foods per week.

Guidelines also include an increased intake of fruits, vegetables, cereals, and grains in a nutrient-rich diet that is low in fat and high in fiber. Multivitamins and other supplements should be used to augment, not replace, natural foods. Pharmacologically manufactured nutrients may not have the same value as those found in nature. As an example, beta-carotene may be more effective when our bodies extract this nutrient from natural foods rather than from synthetic sources. Varieties of fruits and vegetables are necessary. Research has shown the cruciferous vegetables to have a marked effect on incidences of prostate cancer. The **cruciferous vegetables** include broccoli, cauliflower, cabbage, brussel sprouts, bok choy, and kale.

Men who consume more than twenty-eight servings of vegetables weekly have a thirty-five percent decreased risk for prostate cancer compared to men eating fewer than fourteen servings per week.

Carotenoids

There are more than 500 different carotenoids, which are pigments synthesized by plants. They are required for normal cellular growth and differentiation and act as antioxidants. In tissue culture experiments, a variety of carotenoids, including lycopene, accumulate in the prostate and inhibit the growth of prostate cancer cells.

Lycopene

Studies on the Mediterranean diet and the relatively low incidence of prostate cancer in men consuming the diet have led researchers to look closely at the tomato. According to leading cancer specialist Dr. Francisco Contreras, "You've heard the expression *an apple a day . . .* it would be more accurate to say *a tomato a day.*" In his book *A Tomato a Day*, Dr. Contreras goes into great detail on the benefits of lycopene.

The major dietary source of lycopene is cooked and processed tomatoes. A recent study showed that prostate cancer risk was reduced by thirty-five percent in the individuals who consumed greater than ten servings of tomato products per week versus those who consumed fewer than two servings per week. Tomatoes reduce the risk of prostate cancer more than any other food, and the reason must be lycopene.

Does this mean that lycopene can have an effect on men already diagnosed with prostate cancer? In very recent studies, thirty men with prostate adenocarcinoma were recruited and consumed tomato sauce-based pasta dishes for three weeks, roughly the equivalent of 30 mg of lycopene per day. These were all men wishing to avoid a radical prostectomy. Their lycopene levels doubled as a result of dietary supplementation with tomato sauce, and the lycopene levels in their prostate tripled. Moreover, the leukocyte oxidative DNA damage was significantly reduced after the dietary intervention as compared with the levels measured before the tomato sauce was introduced into their diet. Prostate tissue oxidative DNA damage was also statistically lower in men who had the dietary intervention than in randomly selected patients.

Selenium

Selenium is an essential trace nutrient that is critical for the activity of glutathione peroxidase, which protects DNA and other cellular molecules against oxidative damage. In animal testing, high levels have been shown to be protective against some carcinogens. Selenium is found in vegetables and garlic grown in selenium-rich soil. Lower age-specific death rates from some types of cancer are noted in areas with higher selenium levels in the soil. High blood levels of selenium have been associated with decreased risks of cancer in several studies. Some of those studies have looked specifically at prostate cancer.

Scientists at the Stanford University Medical Center conducted a trial to compare blood levels of men with known prostate cancer to the selenium levels in men without prostate cancer. Fifty-two men with prostate cancer were compared to ninety-six men of the same age with no known prostate disease. Some of the men in the group without prostate cancer went on to develop prostate cancer. Blood levels of selenium were recorded for all patients. Those who had the lowest levels of selenium were four to five times more likely to go on to develop prostate cancer than those with the highest levels. Blood levels of selenium were also noted to drop as the men aged, and, of course, prostate cancer risk increases with age.

Vitamin E

Vitamin E is a potent antioxidant that has the ability to inhibit malignant transformation. This fat-soluble vitamin has a powerful effect on the immune system and has been shown to have a substantial protective effect against prostate cancer. The most biologically active and common source of vitamin E is alpha-tocopherol, one of eight naturally occurring forms. The Prostate Cancer Research Institute's recommended dose of vitamin E for patients with prostate cancer is 800-1,200 mg per day. Higher doses of vitamin E are not recommended because they can have blood-thinning effects, which can cause bleeding tendencies. Vitamin E, selenium, and zinc are intimately involved in a number of complementary cellular enzyme systems. Therefore, supplementation with vitamin E should always be done in conjunction with selenium and zinc supplementation. Vitamins E and C also work side by side in antioxidant systems, and supplementation programs should balance these vitamins.

Zinc

Researchers at the University of Maryland initiated a study as a result of the observation that the "normal human prostate accumulates the highest levels of zinc of any soft tissue in the body." From the findings of their study, they concluded that "there now exists strong evidence that the loss of a unique capability to retain a high level of zinc is an important factor in the growth of malignant prostate cells." Men should always ensure that there is enough zinc in their diets since the health of their prostate gland may depend upon it.

> By combining **Ultimate Living Multi-Vitamin** and our **Men's Formula** or by taking the **Daily Health Pack for Men,** you will receive the 30 mg of zinc required for maximum prostate protection.

Vitamin C

Many studies describe the role of vitamin C (ascorbic acid) in protecting against cancer development and in the treatment of established cancer. Due to its importance in the development of immune system cells, vitamin C is crucial as a first line of defense against mutated cells ever multiplying into cancer cells.

Even after the most successful surgery, radiation, or chemotherapy, some cancer cells are bound to remain. It is our immune system that will hunt down these cells and destroy them. Vitamin C is required for our immune systems to generate and mobilize the specialized cells that fight cancer as well as infections. The more stress your immune system is under, the more vitamin C will be used if it is available.

Physicians and researchers differ as to what is considered a therapeutic dosage of vitamin C. If you have prostate cancer and are undergoing treatment, you need to talk to your oncologist regarding dosage.

Vitamin D

A new study suggests that vitamin D may reduce the risk of prostate cancer or at least prevent it from becoming aggressive. Vitamin D is important for calcium metabolism. Dietary vitamin D can be ingested from plant sterols (ergosterol), milk, and foods that have been supplemented with vitamin D. It is also produced by the action of ultraviolet radiation on the skin.

Fiber

Numerous epidemiologic and laboratory studies have indicated a role for dietary fiber during the development and progression of prostate cancer. These epidemiologic studies suggest that the amount of dietary fiber intake could affect prostate cancer by influencing sex steroid production. Fiber from grains, cereals, and nuts is shown to be helpful protection against prostate cancer.

Soy protein

Soy has been in the news recently due to its anti-cancer potential. Soy protein can be found in many foods, including alternatives to meat such as tofu and non-dairy products such as soy yogurts and soy milk. The soybeans from which the protein is extracted contain isoflavanoids. The best known of these is genistein, which has been shown to inhibit prostate cancer cell growth in the laboratory.

Asian men are much less likely to develop clinical cancer than American men. Investigators have linked this difference to the variation in soy protein consumption, which is high in Asian countries. Soy protein consumption is estimated to average 50 g per day in Asian countries compared to less than 2-3 g per day in western diets. In Taiwan, the intake of isoflavones has been shown to be as high as 100 mg per day.

Isoflavones

The importance of isoflavones is widely appreciated and is currently the subject of intense research and discussion. Isoflavones appear to protect against hormone-related disorders such as breast cancer and prostate cancers.

Eating isoflavones-rich products may protect against enlargement of the male prostate gland. Studies show isoflavones slowed prostate cancer growth and caused prostate cancer cells to die. Isoflavones act against cancer cells in a way similar to many common cancer-treatment drugs.

The best way to consume isoflavones is in the form of soy so you can benefit from other healthy components of soy at the same time. The highest amounts of isoflavones can be found in soy nuts and tempeh. Isoflavones are fairly stable. Under normal cooking methods, isoflavones are not destroyed.

For Overall Prostate Health

☆ *Maintain a normal weight for your height.*

☆ *Avoid fatty foods, and try to decrease your fat intake.*

☆ *Eat red meat and processed meat in moderation.*

☆ *Include at least five portions of fruit and vegetables per day, including a regular intake of tomatoes.*

☆ *Include soy products within your diet as an occasional food product.*

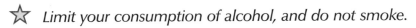 Limit your consumption of alcohol, and do not smoke.

☆ *Protect and strengthen your immune system with good nutrition and effective supplementation.*

☆ *We recommend Ultimate Living Multi-Vitamin and our Men's Formula or our Daily Health Pack for Men for prostate supplementation.*

Heart Disease in Men

Men's risk of having heart disease is higher than women's until women reach menopause.

Major controllable factors that contribute to heart disease are:

- High blood cholesterol levels
- High blood pressure
- Diabetes
- Obesity
- Cigarette smoking
- Physical inactivity

Stress is increasingly a risk factor for heart disease and stroke. Men seem to be particularly vulnerable to stress in the workplace and to financial stresses.

Increasing age and genetics also play key roles in heart disease.

Diet-related recommendations for heart health include the following:

- Reduce the amounts of total fat, saturated fat (found in animal products such as meat, higher fat dairy products, butter, and eggs), trans-fatty acids (found in liquid oils that have been chemically hardened such as margarine, Crisco, and most commercial cookies and baked products), cholesterol, and sodium (salt) in your diet.

- With the guidance of your health-care provider, monitor and control blood pressure and blood cholesterol levels.

- Maintain a healthy weight.

- If you have diabetes, manage your blood glucose levels well.

- Eat plenty of high fiber foods (whole grains; fresh fruits and vegetables; legumes such as beans, peas, and lentils; nuts and seeds). *

- Limit your alcohol intake.

✳ Fruits and Vegetables

Fruits and vegetables are the most important source of antioxidants in our diets. They are especially rich in vitamin C, the carotenes, and the flavonoids. Vitamin E is also found in vegetables; and other good sources are whole-grain cereals, fortified breakfast cereals, and vegetable oils. There is much evidence that suggests that a diet rich in fruits and vegetables protects against heart disease.

Supplements

CoQ10– CoQ10 has been used for years to fight heart disease and to treat the early stages of congestive heart failure in Europe and Japan, and it is now finally gaining mainstream acceptance here in the United States. CoQ10 is beneficial for a broad range of cardiovascular diseases, including hypertension (high blood pressure), congestive heart failure (CHF), and angina. Supplementation with CoQ10 should always be in soft gel form.

Ultimate Living CoQ10 is a softgel formulated to insure maximum bio-availability.

B vitamins– Homocysteine has emerged after twenty-five years of research as the "new cholesterol," and researchers estimate that it is a major risk factor in ten to forty percent of heart attacks and strokes in the United States. Under normal circumstances, this amino acid is short-lived in the system. B vitamin deficiency can prohibit the breakdown of homocysteine.

Ultimate Living B Complex–Lingual includes B-12, B-6, and folic acid. Our B-12 is derived from methylcobalamine, the best source of B-12.

L-Carnitine– supplemental L-carnitine has been well-documented to reduce blood and tissue lipids, a process associated with a reduced risk of developing heart disease.

Ultimate Living Cardio Care contains these valuable nutrients and more for heart protection. Cardio Care is an exclusive blend of herbs, vitamins, enzymes, antioxidants, and amino acids that play a crucial role in heart muscle function.

For more detailed information on nutrition and heart disease, refer to Chapter Seven.

Osteoporosis in Men

Even though the majority of people affected by osteoporosis are women, 20 percent of men are also affected. Today, 2 million American men have osteoporosis, and another 12 million are at risk for this disease. Of the 25 million Americans with osteoporosis, every one in five is a man.

Men need calcium too. When men don't get adequate amounts of dietary calcium, their bodies meet the need by stealing calcium from their bones. This weakens the bones over time and contributes to the development of osteoporosis. Calcium deficiency may also contribute to a number of other medical conditions including hypertension, colon cancer, and tooth loss.

Men need to assure they get adequate calcium and vitamin D everyday.

> *Ultimate Living Cal-Mag Plus* contains hydroxyapatite calcium, the most absorbable form of calcium (ten times more effective than other types of calcium) for the prevention of bone loss. *Cal-Mag Plus* also contains boron and vitamin D for maximum calcium retention. It is very important that calcium and magnesium be in the correct ratio. This means the dosage of magnesium should be exactly half that of calcium. For example, for every 1000 mg of calcium you would need 500 mg of magnesium for maximum benefit.

Resources

Men are less apt to take care of their health than women. In fact, it is often up to the women in their lives to get them to screenings and regular health exams.

More is learned every year about the effects of lifestyle and nutrition on men's special conditions. The American Heart Association, The American Cancer Society, The American Lung Association, The American Diabetes Association, and many others publish specific guidelines for men's health annually.

Chapter Five

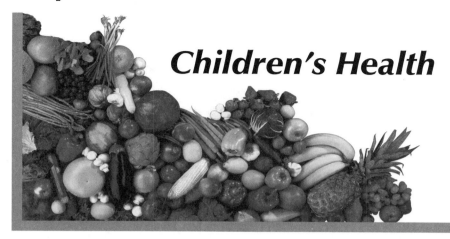

Children's Health

K eeping your child healthy is a big job. By encouraging healthy eating habits and physical activity, you will find that you are making fewer visits to the pediatrician and that your child is missing fewer school days because of minor infections, colds, and flu.

In a country where food is in such ample supply, it is a crime that many of our children go undernourished. We are not discussing children in poverty. These are children of upscale families, the same kids you see shopping in the malls with their mothers and stopping into a fast-food restaurant for a lunch of fattening, empty calories.

Recent studies show that by age six children's arteries are already beginning to show signs of plaque. Our schools are not helping the situation.

Public schools are serving our children meals that lack nutritional value. Lunches include foods such as pizza, French fries, fried shrimp, cheese nachos, and hot pockets. Vegetables are normally limited to one serving per plate and usually consist of corn, mashed potatoes, or, at best, broccoli coated with powdered cheese sauce. Drinks are mostly sugar-loaded fruit drinks, a "healthy" alternative to sodas. Does anyone really think these are appropriate foods for developing minds and bodies?

To insure your child is getting proper nutrition, you should choose a diet with plenty of grain products, vegetables, and fruits. These are all part of a varied diet that provides vitamins, minerals, complex carbohydrates (starch and dietary fiber), and other substances essential for good health and development. Generally these foods are low in fat, depending on their preparation and what is added to them (butter, oils). Nearly all American children are eating far too few servings of grains, vegetables, and fruits even though research shows that consumption of these nutrients is vital to reduce risk for chronic disease.

Kids' Nutrition

Offering children a variety of foods at a young age is the way to allow them to establish good choices early. These include grain products high in complex carbohydrates such as whole-grain breads, cereals, brown rice, and some whole-grain pastas.

Fiber is found only in plant foods; and because there are different kinds of fiber, you should offer your child a variety of plant foods every day— whole grains, beans and peas, and other fruits and vegetables. Fiber is best obtained through foods rather than supplements.

Most fruits and vegetables are naturally low in fat and provide many of the nutrients essential for kids to grow healthy and strong. Plus fruits and vegetables contain valuable antioxidants as well as certain minerals such as potassium and calcium.

Kids need protein, too. Meat, fish, dried beans, eggs, and nuts are all valuable sources of protein. Foods to avoid are hot dogs, luncheon meats, bacon/sausage, peanut butter, and all fried foods.

Water is essential, and children should be encouraged to drink pure, filtered, or natural spring water. If children never start drinking sugary drinks and sodas, they won't want them. As tempting as it is to give in to the begging for a soda, offer an organic fruit juice or low-fat milk instead, and there is always WATER!

Always dilute fruit juice with water to cut down on your child's consumption of sugar (most fruit juices have high sugar content). If you start diluting their juice early, they will never know the difference and will not develop a taste for drinks that are too sweet.

Calcium is important for the development of strong bones and teeth, but dairy should be limited to low-fat or fat free unless the child is younger than two years. Infants and young toddlers need more fat than their older siblings. After the age of two, all children need a complete multivitamin formulated just for kids.

Ultimate Living Multi-Vitamin 4 Kids with Green Miracle provides children with all the nutrients necessary to develop healthy bones and tissues and to ensure mental clarity.

Meal Planning

▷ **Breakfast.** Make sure your child starts his/her day with a nutritious breakfast followed with a good multivitamin. Research shows that children who sit down to a good breakfast perform better in school. A simple yet nutritious breakfast can include fresh fruit, yogurt, and a bowl of cereal.

> **Lunch.** Lunch is the most challenging meal for school-age children. They have access to all the "bad foods" in school cafeterias, vending machines, and friends' lunch bags. Lunch, however, should contain all of the food groups: breads, fruits, vegetables, protein, and dairy. Vary the lunch menus so the child does not become bored and seek out those vending machines and unhealthy school lunches.

> **Dinner.** The most important aspect of dinner should be a designated time for the family to sit down, relax, and talk. What is served on the table will not be as important as what is offered in terms of the quality time with your children. Dinner should be a meal that everyone happily anticipates and enjoys.

To add one more stumbling block to your child's nutrition, our soil has been depleted to the point that valuable nutrients are diminished from most of the food we buy in supermarkets. Organic foods are certainly better; but even if you are preparing all organic foods, a good quality children's multivitamin is necessary to take up the slack.

Attention-Deficit/Hyperactivity Disorder (ADD/ADHD)

Attention-deficit/hyperactivity disorder (ADD or ADHD) is an upsetting and frustrating disease not only for those who have the condition, but also for their friends and relatives as well as the physicians trying to control it. Much of the frustration is due to the exact causes of the condition not being known, which makes treatment options difficult to isolate. This may explain why the current method of treatment is simply to mask the symptoms rather than treat the underlying causes.

It is now known that the drugs historically used—powerful stimulants such as Ritalin, Dexedrine, and Cylert—often do no good and have frequent and sometimes dangerous side effects. Ritalin, for example, is known to cause nervousness and insomnia; and other reactions include skin rashes, fever, weight loss, even hair loss. More seriously, anemia and leucopenia have also been associated with the taking of Ritalin. Dizziness, heart palpitations, cardiac arrhythmia, blood pressure and pulse changes, and angina have all been experienced. These can be terrifying symptoms for a well-adjusted adult. Imagine a child experiencing them.

There is no doubt that the symptoms of ADD will drive parents to seek relief. A child suffering with ADD can wreak havoc on a family.

The symptoms of ADD include:

- Excessive fidgeting, especially with hands and feet

- Difficulty remaining still/seated

- Difficulty following instructions or completing tasks

- Difficulty in playing quietly

- Excessive interrupting of conversations

- Intrusions into other children's play

- Appearing not to understand what is being said–not listening

- Reckless behavior without consideration of the consequences

- Lack of concentration

Adults suffering from the disorder may find themselves with:

- Difficulty in making decisions

- Forgetfulness, being easily distracted

- Lack of concentration

- Hyperactivity

- Impatience

The number of children suffering with learning and behavioral disorders has reached epidemic proportions. These kids have been labeled with ADD, and, unfortunately, those suffering from this disorder may suffer long-term problems in learning and socialization.

> *In addition, studies have shown that children who have taken prescription drugs for ADD have a higher risk of becoming addicted to illegal drugs as a young adult than children who have never taken such drugs.*

Nutrition

As we have said, the causes are basically unknown; but nutritional deficiencies, neurochemical imbalances, food allergies, and hypoglycemia are all suspected. Other factors may be food additives and preservatives, environmental toxins, and poor eating habits. Since food sensitivities play a role in behavioral disorders, affected children should always be tested for food allergens. Children with ADD should avoid foods containing additives, food coloring, preservatives, and sugar.

Essential Fatty Acids

Researchers have found that children with ADD may not be developing correctly due to certain nutritional deficiencies, the most common being EFAs , essential fatty acids.

EFAs are essential because they are vital for proper growth and neurological development. Humans lack the enzymes to produce them. Therefore, they must come from a good diet or from supplementation. EFAs can be found in greatest concentrations in cold water fish such as salmon. Supplements containing fish oil may be beneficial to children and adults suffering from ADD.

A Purdue University study showed that children low in Omega-3 essential fatty acids are significantly more likely to be hyperactive, have learning disorders, and to display behavioral problems. The American diet is almost devoid of Omega-3 except for certain types of fish. In fact, researchers believe that about sixty percent of Americans are deficient in Omega-3 fatty acids, and about twenty percent have so little that test methods cannot even detect any in their blood.

B Vitamins

Several studies have shown that B vitamins may be essential for children with ADD. B vitamins are directly associated with decreased mental performance and are directly responsible for good development of the nervous system, metabolism, and psychiatric health. Vitamins B-6, B-12, and folic acid deficiencies are all associated with behavioral problems as well as with depression and certain psychiatric disorders.

Magnesium

Other research has shown that mineral deficiencies can contribute to ADD. For example, magnesium has been found to be deficient in the blood of children with behavioral problems, and studies have revealed that low magnesium levels are common in hyperactive kids.

Magnesium is a mineral that is needed by every cell of the body. Magnesium is needed for bone, protein, and fatty acid formation; making new cells; activating B vitamins; relaxing muscles; clotting blood; and forming ATP–the muscles' energy source. About half of the body's magnesium stores are found inside the cells of body tissues and organs, and half are combined with calcium and phosphorus in bone. Only one percent of the magnesium in the body is found in blood.

Dietary sources of magnesium include green vegetables such as spinach as well as nuts, seeds, and some whole grains. The magnesium content of refined foods is usually low. Whole-wheat bread, for example, has twice as much magnesium as white bread because the magnesium-rich germ and bran are removed when white flour is processed.

Antioxidants

The powerful antioxidant lipoic acid has been shown to produce positive results in this area. It acts as a cofactor for a number of important enzymes that are responsible for the conversion of food into energy. Clinical studies show that lipoic acid can help to normalize sugar levels in individuals with ADD/ADHD.

The best approach to ADD/ADHD begins with nutrition. Ideally, the diet should be high in vegetable proteins and whole grains and should include plenty of fresh fruits and vegetables. Tryptophan-rich foods, including turkey, fish, wheat germ, and eggs, can have a calming effect. The diet should be supplemented with essential fatty acids and other vital nutrients.

Asthma

Asthma is more common than you might think. As many as five million children in the United States suffer from this disease. Asthma affects about one or two children out of ten. Asthma can start at any age–at infancy through adulthood–but it's most common in school-age children. Asthma flare-ups may sound a little like a cold, with coughing and wheezing.

There are a lot of triggers. Some children are sensitive to allergens – substances that cause allergic reactions in the airways. Common allergens for children with asthma include dust mites, mold, animal dander, and pollen.

Some substances can trigger flare-ups because they irritate the airways and can act just like allergens. These include perfume, chalk dust, and cigarette smoke.

Sometimes an infection can be a trigger and set off an asthma flare-up. If a child comes down with a cold or the flu, his or her airways may become more sensitive than usual. In some children, cold air itself can cause an asthma flare-up and so can exercise.

In between flare-ups, breathing can be totally normal or seem that way. But during a flare-up, it can feel like the person is breathing through a straw. A child with asthma may wheeze (a whistling sound when he or she breathes), cough, and feel tightness in the chest.

Asthma is frightening and can be a dangerous condition. Advances in treatment enable asthma sufferers to avoid attacks and lessen the severity of attacks when they do occur.

Supplements that may be beneficial to relieve asthma symptoms include:

- Magnesium–relaxes constricted bronchial passages and smooth muscles of the throat.

- Vitamin C–acts as an antihistamine to open up constricted airways.

- Quercetin–interferes with several enzyme systems that promote inflammation.

- Ginkgo leaf extract significantly reduces airway hyper-reactivity and improves clinical symptoms and pulmonary functions of asthma patients.

- Zinc is another helpful mineral in the fight against asthma.

*We have received numerous testimonies from parents of children who received relief from breathing difficulties when taking **Ultimate Living Lung Formula**.*

Parental Guidelines

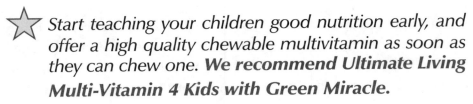 *Start teaching your children good nutrition early, and offer a high quality chewable multivitamin as soon as they can chew one. **We recommend Ultimate Living Multi-Vitamin 4 Kids with Green Miracle.***

☆ *Teach your children the value of good health.*

☆ *Pay careful attention to any changes in your child's behavior and eating or sleeping habits, and alert your pediatrician to anything out of the ordinary.*

☆ *Encourage physical activity and emphasize its value. Children should exercise 60 minutes per day.*

☆ *Offer good food choices and a wide variety of foods.*

☆ *Choose a diet with plenty of grain products, vegetables, and fruits.*

☆ *Choose a diet low in fat, saturated fat, and cholesterol.*

☆ *Choose a diet moderate in sugars and salt.*

☆ *Choose a diet that provides enough calcium and iron to meet the requirements of a growing body.*

☆ *Buy low-calorie and low-fat meals, snacks, and desserts as well as low fat or skim milk.*

☆ *Avoid buying high calorie desserts or snacks such as chips, soft drinks, or ice cream.*

You can also help promote good nutrition by setting a good example. Healthy eating habits and regular exercise should be a consistent part of your family's life. It is much easier if everyone in the house follows these guidelines. Plus you will be instilling lifelong practices that your child will pass on to his or her own family.

Chapter Six

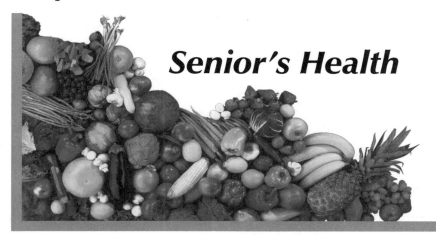

Senior's Health

A ging should not mean illness and dependency. We are all living longer. On the following pages we hope to offer advice on how to live longer and better.

Taking Care of Yourself

The following strategies that have been proven to be effective in promoting the health of older adults are offered by Centers for Disease Control and Prevention and National Center for Chronic Disease Prevention and Health Promotion.

Healthy lifestyles

Research has shown that healthy lifestyles are more influential than genetic factors in helping older people avoid the deterioration traditionally associated with aging. People who are physically active, eat a healthy diet, do not use tobacco, and practice other healthy behaviors including taking nutritional supplements, reduce their risk for chronic diseases and have half the rate of disability of those who do not.

Early detection of diseases

Screening to detect chronic diseases early in their course, when they are most treatable, can save many lives; however, many older adults have not had recommended screenings. For example, sixty percent of Americans over age 65 have not had a sigmoidoscopy or colonoscopy in the previous five years to screen for colorectal cancer even though Medicare covers the cost.

Immunizations

More than 40,000 people age 65 or older die each year of influenza and invasive pneumococcal disease. Immunizations reduce a person's risk of hospitalization and death from these diseases. Yet in 2002, thirty-two percent of Americans age 65 or older had not had a recent flu shot, and thirty-seven percent had never received a pneumonia vaccine.

Injury prevention

Falls are the most common cause of injuries to older adults. More than one-third of adults age 65 or older fall each year; and of those who fall, twenty to thirty percent suffer moderate to severe injuries that decrease mobility and independence. Removing tripping hazards in the home and installing grab bars are simple measures that can greatly reduce older Americans' risk for falls and fractures.

Self-management techniques

Programs to teach older Americans self-management techniques can reduce both the pain and costs of chronic disease. For example, the Arthritis Self-Help Course, disseminated by the Arthritis Foundation, has been shown to reduce arthritis pain by twenty percent and visits to physicians by forty percent. Unfortunately, less than one percent of Americans with arthritis participate in such programs, and courses are not available in many areas.

Physical Activity

Physical activity strengthens muscles and bones. Since falls account for many disabilities in seniors, exercising regularly and remaining physically active reduce the chances for serious injury. You should always talk to your physician before starting an exercise program, and he or she will offer advice on the right form of exercise for you based on your level of fitness.

Free weights are an excellent form of exercise to retain or regain strength and to help prevent osteoporosis.

Dietary Recommendations

Add dietary fiber to your diet. Doing this one thing alone is a positive step towards better health as you age.

Foods high in fiber include:

- Unprocessed wheat bran
- Unrefined breakfast cereals
- Whole wheat and rye flours
- Grainy breads such as whole wheat, rye, or pumpernickel
- Fresh organic fruits such as apples and berries
- Dried fruits such as prunes, apricots, and figs
- Organic vegetables such as broccoli and carrots
- Legumes such as chickpeas, baked beans, and lima beans

Supplements for Senior Complaints

It is always best to talk to your health care provider and/or pharmacist who are familiar with the medications you are taking before starting any supplements or herbal remedies.

Multiple vitamin–a good, natural multivitamin is needed to fill in your dietary gaps.

Coenzyme Q10 is a naturally occurring antioxidant that exists in all human cells. CoQ10 is beneficial in the prevention of cardiovascular disease. Ongoing research has shown that its use may slow the functional decline of patients with Parkinson's disease.

Vitamin E is a naturally occurring vitamin essential for human life. It is commonly considered a skin conditioner, antioxidant, heart protector, and memory enhancer. Research is ongoing about the use of this vitamin for the treatment and prevention of Alzheimer's disease.

> *Ultimate Living Multi-Vitamin is a good nutritional value containing much needed nutrients plus 400 IU of vitamin E.*

Calcium is a mineral found in bones and teeth. Reduced absorption of calcium can lead to osteoporosis in older people.

Dehydroepiandrosterone (DHEA) is a hormone produced by the human adrenal glands. DHEA supplements are often touted as a way to reverse the effects of aging by boosting immunity, improving memory, and increasing muscle mass. DHEA supplementation should always be approved by your doctor.

Saw palmetto is the oily extract of the berries from the saw palmetto, a type of palm tree. It is primarily used to improve urinary flow associated with an enlarged prostate. An enlarged prostate can signal more serious conditions such as prostate cancer. Consult your physician if you are having urinary difficulties.

Glucosamine is a natural component of joint cartilage. Glucosamine and chondroitin act as natural anti-inflammatory agents to relieve the pain, swelling, and stiffness of arthritis. When coupled with Green-Lipped mussel, the dual action formula is particularly effective.

*Ultimate Living Arthritis Formula contains the effective combination of glucosamine and chondroitin with the added benefit of Green-Lipped mussel as well as other valuable nutrients. Our **Arthritis Formula** provides excellent nutritional support for bones, joints, ligaments, and other connective tissues and can provide relief from pain, swelling, and stiffness.*

Ginkgo leaf extract may act as a memory enhancer and treatment for Alzheimer's disease. People with clotting disorders need to check with their physician before taking any form of ginkgo.

St. John's wort may elevate mood and act as an anti-depressant. It may alleviate mild to moderate depression and related anxiety and insomnia. St. John's wort should not, however, take the place of counseling in these cases.

Kava is commonly used to relieve anxiety and has also been used as an anticonvulsant. It is dangerous in conjunction with alcohol, sedatives, or antipsychotic drugs.

Beware of natural formulas touted as "natural Viagra." They may contain ma huang (a Chinese stimulant) that has been linked to stroke, heart attack, and death.

Maintaining Independence

Eating a healthy, fiber-rich diet, exercising regularly, and participating in your community should enable you to remain independent for a long time. The main factor in staying independent is staying well. Hopefully the information provided in these pages will help you do so.

Everyone wants to maintain independence and not to have to resort to depending on others. There may be times, however, when you do need a hand. Asking for help can be difficult. Think about it. At some point your children or others relied upon you for help. Don't be afraid to ask them for help when you need it. Talk to your doctor, family, or community organizations and agencies about what other services or options might be available to meet your needs. Be willing to ask for what you need.

Chapter Seven

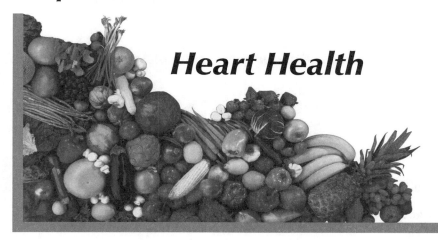

Heart Health

A lmost six million hospitalizations each year in the United States are due to cardiovascular disease. Every 20 seconds a person in the United States has a heart attack. Every 34 seconds a person in the United States dies from heart disease. At least 250,000 people die of heart attacks each year before they reach a hospital. Awareness of one's own risk factors, knowledge of warning signs, medical intervention, and, most important, a healthy lifestyle can be crucial in surviving or avoiding heart disease!

An average heart pumps 2.4 ounces (70 milliliters) per heartbeat. An average heartbeat is 72 beats per minute. Therefore, an average heart pumps 1.3 gallons (5 liters) per minute. In other words, it pumps 1,900 gallons (7,200 liters) per day, almost 700,000 gallons (2,628,000 liters) per year, or 48 million gallons (184,086,000 liters) by the time someone is 70 years old. That's a lot of hard work!

Heart disease is not an obvious illness. People who have this disease can walk around looking and feeling perfectly healthy. For many, a heart attack is the first sign of heart disease. But it does not have to be this way, and when it comes to surviving heart disease, the most important factor is an early diagnosis.

Risk Factors

All of us need to be aware of our specific risk factors which include:

- A family history of heart disease
- Low HDL
- High blood pressure
- High blood sugar
- Excess weight
- Cigarette smoking
- Male over 45
- Female over 55 or after menopause
- Lack of exercise–inactivity
- High stress environment
- Elevated homocysteine levels
- Plaque in coronary arteries

In addition, research is providing much new information that allows doctors to see early warning signs. For example, evidence is growing that chronic **inflammation** of the arteries, a painless condition, weakens the arterial walls and can cause fatty build-ups to burst. Inflammation can be caused by a number of things, including smoking. Researchers are associating bacterial infections such as gum disease, chronic bladder infections, and viruses with the onset of heart disease. Doctors are now able to use a simple blood test called CRP (Creatine Reactive Protein) to measure for a protein produced by the body's efforts to fight infection.

This new focus on the dangers of chronic inflammation underlines the importance of keeping the immune system running at its best and may also throw light on why antioxidants seem to play a positive role in preventing coronary disease.

Free radicals can damage the heart and blood vessels, and we know that antioxidants are free radicals' natural enemy. It would follow that a diet rich in antioxidants would be beneficial in preventing heart disease. The most recognized dietary antioxidants are vitamin C, vitamin E, selenium, and carotenoids.

Family History

Some families seem to be genetically predisposed to heart disease. If this is your case, you must address all of the other risk factors in order to give yourself the best chance to avoid heart disease. These are discussed in the sections that follow.

Homocysteine

Great attention is now being paid to homocysteine, an amino acid. Evidence shows that its presence in the bloodstream is linked to an increased risk of heart disease due to inflammation. High levels of homocysteine damage the arterial walls and make it easier for cholesterol to build up in the arteries. Homocysteine actually acts like a corrosive acid on the arterial walls. Too much of it is related to a higher risk of coronary heart disease, stroke, and peripheral vascular disease (fatty deposits in peripheral arteries). Evidence suggests that homocysteine may promote atherosclerosis (fatty deposits in blood vessels) by damaging the inner lining of arteries and promoting blood clots. Homocysteine levels in the blood are strongly influenced by diet and genetic factors.

Studies have found that higher blood levels of B vitamins are related to lower concentrations of homocysteine. Other evidence indicates that low blood levels of folic acid are linked with a higher risk of fatal coronary heart disease and stroke. Folic acid and other B vitamins help break down homocysteine in the body. Persons at risk for heart disease should be sure to get enough folic acid and vitamins B-6 and B-12 in their diet. They should eat at least five servings of fruits and green leafy vegetables daily. The combination of B-12, B-6, and folic acid can be most effective in lowering elevated homocysteine levels that contribute to stroke as well as cardiovascular disease. Also, to produce CoQ10, your body needs B vitamins and folic acid.

> *A combination of **Ultimate Living B Complex-Lingual** and **Ultimate Living CoQ10** will help to protect against a build-up of homocysteine.*

Cholesterol

High cholesterol remains one of the big risks for heart disease although medicine has come a long way in getting people to lower their cholesterol through diet and exercise.

> *Drinking green tea has been linked with a lowered risk of cancer, lower cholesterol, anti-aging, weight loss, and even diabetes prevention.*

Cholesterol levels have long been thought to contribute to coronary disease. Most people do not understand the results of their cholesterol screenings. The total cholesterol is a measurement of the total amount of cholesterol in your bloodstream.

➤ High density lipoprotein (HDL) or "good cholesterol" helps clear excess lipids from the arteries. The higher this number is the better. An HDL of 60 mg/dl or more is helpful. An HDL of 40 mg/dl or less is considered a risk factor for heart disease.

➤ The TC/HDL ratio is a comparison of total cholesterol to your HDL. A ratio of 4.5 or less is desirable. The lower the ratio, the less risk you have of developing heart disease.

➤ Low density lipoprotein (LDL), or "bad cholesterol," contributes to the build-up of fat deposits on the arterial walls. Approximately 65 percent of the cholesterol in your blood is LDL. An LDL of less than 130 mg/dl is desirable. If you have a personal history of coronary disease, physicians like to see your LDL below 100 mg/dl, and some suggest 70 mg/dl as a goal for those at high risk.

Triglycerides are composed of fatty acids and glycerol. Like cholesterol, they circulate in your blood but are actually stored in body fat. Every time you eat, your triglyceride and glucose levels increase significantly; but if your body processes fat efficiently, the level of triglycerides will decrease. Authorities recommend that triglyceride levels be below 150 mg/dl. The effect of eating on these levels is the reason for fasting before the test.

A lipid profile is a more detailed measure of the fats in your bloodstream. It consists of measuring your total cholesterol, HDL, LDL, and triglycerides and calculating your TC/HDL ratio. Your physician should recommend a lipid profile if your total cholesterol (a simple blood test that does not require fasting) is elevated or if you have other risk factors such as low HDL, a family history of heart disease, high blood pressure, smoking, or diabetes.

HDL and LDL levels are definitely affected by diet and exercise. It is important to consume foods high in fiber such as grains, fruits, vegetables, beans, and legumes and to limit your intake of foods high in saturated fat such as butter, meat, nuts, cream, and egg yolks. The American Heart Association offers excellent information on dietary changes you can make that will positively affect your cholesterol levels.

Plaque in Coronary Arteries

Physicians can detect plaque build-up with new imaging technology and take measures to remove build-up and prevent additional clogging. A diet rich in antioxidants and in whole grains such as oatmeal, wheat germ, and flax seems to offer help in preventing clogged arteries.

High Blood Pressure (hypertension)

High blood pressure is a major health problem in the United States, where, according to the U.S. Centers for Disease Control, more than 50 million people over age sixty (and one in four adults) have the condition. It is especially common among African-Americans, who are one of the most likely ethnic groups in the world to be diagnosed with high blood pressure. It has also been diagnosed in two-thirds of Americans over 65 and a growing number of young adults and children.

High blood pressure is a condition commonly associated with narrowing of the arteries. This causes blood to be pumped with excessive force against the artery walls. It is a sign that the heart and blood vessels are being overworked. Untreated, high blood pressure will cause the heart to eventually overwork itself to the point where serious damage can occur.

High blood pressure is known as the "silent killer" because it often goes undetected. Regular exercise, stress reduction, and lowering your intake of sodium (salt) will help lower blood pressure. If yours is elevated, you should be monitoring it regularly. There are numerous, inexpensive blood pressure monitors on the market today. A good way to check the accuracy of your monitor is to take it with you to your doctor and have your blood pressure checked on your monitor as well as on your doctor's.

High Blood Sugar

High blood sugar is a heart-disease risk factor. The most life-threatening consequences of diabetes are heart disease and stroke, which strike people with diabetes more than twice as often as they do others. Most of the cardiovascular complications related to diabetes have to do with the way the heart pumps blood through the body. Diabetes can change the chemical makeup of some of the substances found in the blood, and this can cause blood vessels to narrow or to clog completely. This is called atherosclerosis, or hardening of the arteries, and diabetes seems to speed it up.

The risk of cardiovascular disease among people with diabetes is dramatic. A diagnosis of diabetes as an adult presents the same risk as already having had one heart attack. More than 65 percent of deaths in diabetes patients are attributed to heart and vascular disease.

If you have elevated blood-sugar levels or have been diagnosed with diabetes, it is essential that you control these levels. Diet is a factor; sweets and starchy foods are the culprits. If you are diabetic, you already know to avoid these foods. It is imperative that you control your diabetes. If your doctor has told you that your blood sugar levels are elevated, you may be able to stave off diabetes by controlling your diet, getting proper exercise, and avoiding stress.

Overweight

Being overweight is a contributor to heart disease on many fronts. People who are carrying too much weight tend to be more sedentary than slender people, and we already know that inactivity is a risk factor in heart disease. Overweight people are likely to be eating a diet high in fat. Plus, obesity is a major risk factor in diabetes. There are simply no benefits to being overweight. We will discuss safe weight loss in Chapter Fourteen.

Smoking

If you are still smoking, QUIT! Your physician will offer good advice on the best methods to break this deadly habit.

Aging

Both men and women become more vulnerable to heart disease as they age, but this tends to happen about ten years earlier in men. Statistics show that heart attacks are more prevalent in men after the age of 45 while for women the age is 55 or after menopause. There is nothing we can do about aging; it is a natural part of life. But we can age and maintain good health by implementing good lifestyle practices: healthy diets, good supplementation, low stress, and as much relaxation as possible.

Inactivity

Exercise has a positive effect on the body in general but particularly in relation to the cardiovascular system. Regular exercise is helpful in lowering blood pressure and cholesterol, increasing circulation, maintaining a normal weight, and eliminating stress.

Stress

More and more evidence suggests a relationship between the risk of cardiovascular disease and environmental and psychosocial factors such as job strain, isolation, and personality traits. Research is ongoing to establish how stress contributes to heart disease risk. It is uncertain as to whether or not stress is an independent risk factor, but it is known that stress is extremely debilitating to our health in general.

The good news is that you can lower your risks of having a heart attack by making positive lifestyle changes:

➤ *Eat a heart-healthy diet (The American Heart Association provides excellent dietary information)*

➤ *Get plenty of exercise*

➤ *Maintain proper weight*

➤ *Stop smoking*

➤ *Avoid stress. Keep a healthy balance between work, family, and rest.*

➤ *Do not let diseases such as high blood pressure and diabetes go untreated.*

Adopt a Healthy Eating Plan

It seems that everyone is looking for the magic diet. The bookstore shelves are loaded with books extolling the healthy virtues of everything from low carbohydrates and high protein to high fat intake. But as you have already read, these diets can be extremely detrimental to your heart and cardiovascular system. Yo-yo dieting (continuously losing and gaining weight) has also been shown to be damaging.

A five year study known as the Lyon Heart Diet Study found that there may be no better diet than the "Mediterranean" diet. This diet includes whole-wheat pasta, lentils, asparagus, broccoli, spinach, cabbage, onions, garlic, cherries, peaches, plums, kiwi fruit, fatty fish such as salmon, olive oil, and feta cheese.

Following a good eating plan will help you achieve and maintain a desired weight. The benefits will be a desirable blood cholesterol level and lowered blood pressure. In general, you should always eat plenty of organic vegetables, fruits, whole grains, unprocessed oils, legumes (beans and soy), fatty fish such as salmon, and limited quantities of lean meats. Eliminate fried, greasy, fatty foods from your diet. Get your fats from olive and other pure oils. Eat a variety of organic fruits and vegetables, choosing at least nine servings each and every day. Eat a variety of whole-grain products. Include fat-free and low-fat milk products, fish, legumes, skinless poultry, and lean meats. Choose fats and oils with two grams or less of saturated fat per tablespoon. Replace butter or margarine with olive oil whenever possible.

> *Olive oil has been shown to lower LDL cholesterol. Using two tablespoons of olive oil per day in place of other fats may be enough to produce this LDL lowering effect.*

Balance the number of calories you eat with the number you use each day. To find this number, multiply the number of pounds you weigh by fifteen calories. This represents the average number of calories you use on a moderately active day. If you are sedentary, multiply by thirteen. Maintain a level of physical activity that keeps you fit and matches the number of calories you consume.

Limit your intake of high-caloric foods or foods that are low in nutrition such as soft drinks and candy. Limit foods high in saturated fats and cholesterol such as whole milk products, fatty meats, tropical oils, partially hydrogenated oils, and egg yolks.

Eat less than six grams of salt per day (2,400 milligrams of sodium).

Limit your intake of alcohol.

Recipe for a Healthy Heart

- Eat plenty of vegetables, fruits, whole grains, unprocessed oils, legumes (beans and soy), fatty fish such as salmon, and limited quantities of lean meats.

- Eliminate fried, greasy, fatty foods from your diet. Get your fats from olive and other pure oils.

- Do not buy into fad dieting. High protein/high fat diet regimens contain too much saturated fat, and they contain literally no fiber or phytonutrients that are found in fruits and vegetables.

> ***Ultimate Living Green Miracle*** *is packed with valuable phytonutrients and provides the daily requirement of fruits and vegetables.*

- Adopt a sensible supplementation program.

- Exercise regularly. Regular exercise fills the bloodstream with cleansing oxygen and flushes toxins and wastes from the system.

- De-stress! The heart and cardiovascular system can become severely damaged from chronically high blood pressure brought on by stress. Adrenalin, the body's major stress hormone, causes damage to the lining of the arteries.

- Get plenty of rest and sufficient sleep.

- Breathe! Most Americans are shallow breathers. Learn how to breathe from your diaphragm. Fill your lungs and exhale completely.

Supplementation for Heart Health

CoQ10

CoQ10 or coenzyme Q10 is a powerful antioxidant found throughout the body. The body's store of CoQ10 diminishes with age. In fact, the body's store of CoQ10 peaks at around age twenty and then declines fairly rapidly. Experts involved in CoQ10 research believe that older people are deficient in CoQ10 and would benefit from supplementation.

CoQ10 has been studied extensively in this country since the late 1950s. Since then many scientific studies have shown the clinical efficacy of CoQ10 for preventing and treating cardiovascular disease, including congestive heart failure, coronary heart disease, heart valve disease, rheumatic heart disease, and arrhythmia. CoQ10 has been shown to be effective in periodontal (gum) disease, which, as indicated earlier, is known to be a contributing factor in heart disease.

There are many reasons that the body's production of CoQ10 is hampered. Vitamin and mineral deficiencies can inhibit the natural production of this valuable nutrient. The statin drugs used to lower cholesterol can block the synthesis of CoQ10. Recent research is also reporting that some of the cytotoxic drugs such as Adriamycin, used to treat cancer and a variety of autoimmune illnesses, may induce CoQ10 depletion and increase the risk of cardiovascular disease. Psychotropic drugs, including some antidepressants and beta-blockers, as well as the blood thinning drug coumadin have also been reported to inhibit CoQ10 production.

Between 10 mg and 30 mg per day of CoQ10 is the recommended dose for healthy individuals, but doses for persons taking the statin drugs or cancer patients may need to be higher. The safety of CoQ10 has been well documented by many major studies showing it to have very infrequent side effects.

> *A one-two punch is the combination of CoQ10, beta-carotene, and vitamin E. Beta-carotene helps in the absorption of CoQ10 while vitamin E slows down oxidation. The combination can be very effective in fighting free-radical damage.*

Grape seed and grape seed extract

Grape seed and grape seed extract contain **proanthocyanidins** and are potent antioxidants. Proanthocyanidins are a class of nutrients belonging to the flavonoids. They are found in the skins of fruits and vegetables and are thought to be twenty times more potent in their antioxidant abilities than vitamin C and fifty times more potent than vitamin E. Grape seed extract is a cardio-protector. It gobbles up free radicals and inhibits free radical cell damage. It can help to lower blood pressure and regulate sugar levels.

Vitamin E

Vitamin E can reduce the incidence of such heart disease symptoms as angina and can lower the incidence of coronary artery disease. Although minimal amounts of vitamin E can be obtained through foods such as seeds, nuts, and grains, obtaining maximum antioxidant effects from vitamin E might require the ingestion of too much fat. Vitamin E supplementation is a healthier alternative.

Fish oils

Fish oils appear to reduce the risk of cardiovascular disease since they increase blood clotting time, are effective at reducing LDL, and can reduce inflammation. Research indicates that fish oil helps to provide nutritional support for healthy cardiovascular function as well as for joints and skin. Fish oils may also reduce the severity of arthritis symptoms. The most beneficial fish are cold water fish such as mackerel, herring, salmon, tuna, and sardines. There are numerous fish oil supplements on the market; but just as in selecting fish for dinner, you want to choose one that is natural, stable, and from cold water fish.

Most adults benefit from supplementation of these fatty acids if they are not on a diet that is already rich in fish. In 1999, a study conducted in Italy found that Omega-3 fish oil can reduce the risk of heart-related deaths by thirty percent in people who have suffered heart attacks.

Selenium

Selenium is a trace mineral that is essential to good health but <u>required only in small amounts</u>. Selenium is incorporated into proteins to make selenoproteins, which are important antioxidant enzymes. The antioxidant properties of selenoproteins help prevent cellular damage from free radicals. Plant foods are the major dietary sources of selenium. The content of selenium in food depends on the selenium content of the soil where plants are grown or animals are raised. Selenium can also be found in some meats and seafood. Animals that eat grains or plants grown in selenium-rich soil have higher levels of selenium in their muscle. In the U.S., meats and bread are common sources of dietary selenium. Some nuts are also sources of selenium.

People with acute severe illness who develop inflammation and wide-spread infection often have decreased levels of selenium in their blood. Selenium is an antioxidant that may help limit the oxidation of LDL cholesterol, thereby helping to prevent coronary artery disease.

Some other natural cardio-assists are listed below.

- **Alpha lipoic acid** is an aggressive free-radical fighter that works to promote healthy cardiovascular tissue.

- **Chlorophyll**, the green pigment in all green foods, delivers critically needed oxygen to heart cells.

- **Chromium** is a mineral that plays a valuable role in the regulation of blood sugar, which is essential in preventing the destruction of collagen in the arterial connective tissues.

- **Garlic** has been a natural medicinal powerhouse for centuries. It contains active compounds that effectively reduce cholesterol levels and has been known to help lower blood pressure.

- **L-Carnitine** is an amino acid that speeds up the conversion of glucose to energy in heart cells.

- **Magnesium** reduces blood pressure by relaxing arteries, thus preventing heart and arterial spasms.

- **Niacin** effectively lowers LDL cholesterol. Some people experience an uncomfortable flush when taking large doses of niacin; however, it has long been considered an excellent natural form of cholesterol reduction.

- **Potassium** helps the arterial walls to dilate, therefore lowering blood pressure.

- **Soy** contains isoflavones that are powerful antioxidants with plant sterols capable of replacing LDL cholesterol in cell membranes.

- **Bioperine**, a black pepper extract, helps enhance the absorption of nutrients and increases the effectiveness of CoQ10.

- **Trimethylglycine**, an amino acid, is important in preventing heart disease, stroke, and liver disease.

- **Taurine**, the most abundant amino acid found in the body, is thought to be important in the regulation of the central nervous system.

- **Quercetin**, found in vegetables, fruit skins, and onions, is the most potent flavonoid. Recent studies have demonstrated that flavonoids may act as antioxidants. Diets high in flavonoids have been shown to reduce the risk of heart attack by 68 percent and stroke by as much as 78 percent.

The World Health Organization has highlighted that a diet low or lacking in fruit and vegetable consumption may be a cause of coronary heart disease.

Recognizing Danger Signals

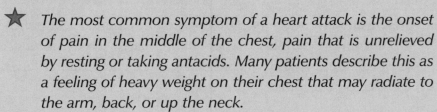 The most common symptom of a heart attack is the onset of pain in the middle of the chest, pain that is unrelieved by resting or taking antacids. Many patients describe this as a feeling of heavy weight on their chest that may radiate to the arm, back, or up the neck.

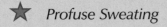 Profuse Sweating

Nausea

Weakness and/or shortness of breath

A sense of "impending doom"

Fifty percent of all heart attack patients will experience all of these symptoms while others may not. The best protection is prevention and detection. If you or someone you are with has these signals, don't wait longer than a few minutes before seeking medical help.

The warning signs of stroke differ greatly from those of a heart attack. They may include sudden numbness or weakness in the face, arm, or leg (especially limited to only one side of the body); sudden confusion; trouble speaking or understanding; sudden trouble seeing in one or both eyes; sudden trouble walking; dizziness; loss of balance or coordination; or sudden, severe headache for no known reason.

Whether a person is having a stroke or a heart attack, calling 9-1-1 is the fastest way to get lifesaving treatment. They can begin medical treatment immediately upon arrival. Remember, patients who arrive at the hospital by ambulance are usually treated more quickly.

Terms You May Need To Know

In the event that you or a loved one is diagnosed with heart disease, these are terms that you might need to know:

Arteriosclerosis: a term covering a series of diseases in which the walls of the arteries thicken and lose their elasticity, commonly referred to as "hardening of the arteries."

Atherosclerosis: the build up of fatty deposits in the innermost layer of the artery wall. It is the most common form of arteriosclerosis in the United States.

Arrhythmia: irregularity or loss of rhythm of the heartbeat.

Cardiac catheterization: passage of a catheter into the heart through a blood vessel leading to the heart. The test is performed for the purpose of measuring intracardiac pressure abnormalities, obtaining cardiac blood samples, and/or imaging cardiac structures by injection of radio-opaque dye.

Catheter: a hollow, cylindrical medical device used for diagnostic or therapeutic purposes.

Coronary artery disease (CAD): atherosclerosis (abnormal hardening/thickening) of the coronary arteries, which may cause angina pectoris, myocardial infarction (heart attack), and sudden death. Both genetically determined and avoidable risk factors contribute to CAD. They include hypercholesterolemia (excessive levels of cholesterol in the blood), hypertension (high blood pressure), smoking, diabetes mellitus, and low levels of high-density lipoproteins.

Coronary stenosis: narrowing or constriction of any orifices leading into or from the heart or between the chambers of the heart.

Coronary thrombus: a blood clot that obstructs a blood vessel of the heart.

Electrocardiogram (ECG or EKG): the major diagnostic tool for evaluating patients with stable angina, unstable angina, myocardial ischemia, or abnormal heart rhythms. The ECG records electrical activity in the heart from various perspectives. Certain changes in this activity are characteristic of myocardial ischemia, infarction, or arrhythmias.

Hypercholesterolemia: the state of having excessive amounts of cholesterol in the blood. Hypercholesterolemia is a risk factor for atherosclerosis.

Hypertension: elevated blood pressure. Hypertension is a risk factor for atherosclerosis.

Infarction: a sudden insufficiency of blood supply leading to death of tissue.

Ischemia: inadequate circulation of blood to a given tissue. When ischemia is sufficiently severe, it can result in infarction.

Ischemic heart disease (IHD): a form of heart disease whose primary manifestations result from myocardial ischemia (ischemia = deficient supply of oxygenated blood) due to atherosclerotic CAD. The term can encompass a spectrum of patients, ranging from the asymptomatic preclinical phase to acute myocardial infarction and sudden cardiac death.

Myocardial infarction: damage to the heart muscle caused by occlusion of one or more of the coronary arteries.

Myocardial ischemia (MI): a condition in which oxygen delivery to, and waste removal from, the myocardium falls below normal levels, with oxygen demand exceeding supply. As a consequence, the metabolic machinery of myocardial cells becomes impaired, leading to various degrees of systolic (contractile) and diastolic (relaxation) dysfunction.

Non-Q-wave myocardial infarction: an acute myocardial infarction that is not associated with the evolution of new Q waves on the ECG. The diagnosis of non-Q-wave myocardial infarction is often difficult to make soon after the event and is commonly established only retrospectively on the basis of elevated cardiac enzyme levels.

Plaque: the pathologic lesion of atherosclerosis. Atherosclerotic plaques contain cholesterol, cellular elements, and connective tissue.

Post-MI angina: unstable angina occurring from one to 60 days after an acute MI.

Restenosis: the recurrence of a stenosis in a coronary artery.

Stenosis: a pathologic narrowing of a tubular structure such as a blood vessel.

Stent: a device inserted into a tubular structure (such as a coronary artery) to prevent that structure from closing.

Thrombus: a blood clot.

Thrombolysis: breaking apart of a thrombus. Thrombolysis can occur physiologically (that is, without intervention) or subsequent to administration of a thrombolytic drug such as t-PA or streptokinase.

Unstable angina: chest pain that occurs at rest, new onset of pain with exertion, or pain that has accelerated (i.e., more frequent, longer in duration, or lower in threshold).

Chapter Eight

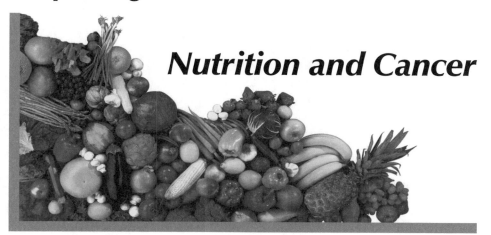

Nutrition and Cancer

C ancer has outpaced heart disease as the number one killer of Americans under the age of 85. It is estimated that approximately one third of all cancers are related to smoking and another third to diet, exercise, and obesity.

Recent information from the American Cancer Society indicates the following:

- The most common type of cancer is non-melanoma skin cancer with more than 1,000,000 new cases expected in the United States in 2005. Non-melanoma skin cancers represent about half of all cancers diagnosed in this country.

- For 2005, the estimated number of new cases of colon cancer is 104,950, and the estimated number of new cases of rectal cancer is 40,340, a slight decrease from the 2004 statistics.

- The total number of new leukemia cases estimated for 2005 is slightly higher than the number estimated for 2004.

- Lung cancer is diagnosed in an estimated 164,000 Americans each year.

● It is estimated that approximately 232,000 men will be diagnosed with prostate cancer in 2005. (Prostate cancer is discussed in detail in Chapter Two)

● Over 211,000 women are expected to be diagnosed with breast cancer in 2005. (Breast cancer is discussed in detail in Chapter Three)

Skin Cancer

Skin cancer, generally a result of overexposure to the sun, is the most commonly diagnosed form of cancer in America. While skin cancers are the most common form of cancer, many types are both preventable and treatable.

Skin cancer is classified into five different types:

▷ Basal cell carcinoma (BCC) is the most common form and accounts for seventy-five percent of all skin cancers. It originates in the basal cells at the bottom of the epidermis (outer skin layer) and is caused by long-term exposure to sunlight.

▷ Squamous cell carcinoma (SCC) is the second most common type, accounting for twenty percent of all skin cancers. It originates in the epidermis, eventually penetrating the underlying tissue if not treated. In a small percentage of cases, this cancer metastasizes, or spreads, to other parts of the body.

▷ Malignant melanoma (MM) is a form of skin cancer that currently is affecting an increasing number of people. There are more than 40,000 new cases of malignant melanoma annually in the U.S., resulting in more than 7,000 deaths. MM is a very serious type of skin cancer, but the cure rate is quite good if it is diagnosed and removed early. MM originates in moles or other growths on normal skin.

▷ Paget's disease (PD) is a rare type of skin cancer. It generally appears on the nipple and is associated with an underlying breast cancer. It may also appear in the groin or near the anus, possibly originating in the sweat glands.

▷ Kaposi's sarcoma (KS) is caused by a virus in the herpes family. An aggressive AIDS-related form affects about one third of AIDS patients. A form that grows more slowly occurs in elderly men of Italian or Jewish ancestry.

Signs and Symptoms

Skin cancer is accompanied by the following signs and symptoms:

★ *New skin lesions or open sores that bleed, ooze, or crust and fail to heal in an expected time frame*

★ *Enlargement of an existing skin lesion*

★ *Change in color of a mole*

★ *Reddish patch or irritated area, frequently occurring on the chest, shoulders, arms, or legs*

★ *Shiny bump that is pearly or translucent*

★ *Poorly defined borders of a skin lesion*

People at Risk

People with the following conditions or characteristics are at risk for developing skin cancer:

- Light skin color

- Spending a lot of time outdoors in work and/or leisure activities

- History of severe sunburn

- Family history of skin cancer

- Large dark-colored birthmark known as congenital melanocytic nevus

- Certain non-cancerous skin conditions, such as actinic keratosis, can predispose a person to skin cancer

- HIV (human immunodeficiency virus) increases the risk of contracting KS

Prevention

Most skin cancers are preventable. If you are in a high-risk category, take measures to avoid sun exposure; and when in the sun, protect yourself by covering up, wearing a hat, and applying sunscreen with an SPF of at least 30.

Nutrition for Skin Cancer

Foods including fish, beans, carrots, chard, pumpkin, cabbage, broccoli, and vegetables containing beta-carotene and vitamin C are all thought to be beneficial in preventing skin cancer. Lignans, substances found in foods such as soy and flaxseed, may also be beneficial in fighting cancer in general, including the spread of melanoma from one part of the body. Green tea contains polyphenols, compounds that are potent antioxidants. The main polyphenol in green tea is epigallocatechin gallate (EGCG). Scientific studies suggest that EGCG and green tea polyphenols may prevent the onset and growth of skin tumors.

See your health care provider regularly for screenings to check for and prevent recurrence of skin cancer.

Colon Cancer

Colorectal cancer is diagnosed in more than 130,000 people each year in the U.S. alone. In the early stages, colorectal cancer can be without noticeable symptoms, so it is important to have regular colorectal screenings to detect early problems.

Symptoms

Not all colorectal cancers are without symptoms. One of the early symptoms of colon cancer may be bleeding. Tumors frequently bleed only small amounts, and evidence of the blood is found only during chemical testing of the stool. When tumors have grown larger, other symptoms may develop.

They include:

> **Change in bowel habits.** Constipation, diarrhea, and bowel incontinence, although usually symptoms of other, less serious problems, can also indicate colorectal cancer.

➤ **Blood on or in the stool.** By far the most alarming of all the symptoms, blood on or in the stool can be a symptom of colorectal cancer. But it does not necessarily indicate cancer. Numerous other problems can cause bleeding in the digestive tract, including hemorrhoids, ulcers, ulcerative colitis, and Crohn's disease, to name only a few. In addition, iron and some foods, such as beets, can give the stool a black or red appearance, falsely indicating blood in the stool. However, if you notice blood in your stool, see your doctor to rule out a serious condition.

➤ **Unexplained anemia.** Anemia is a shortage of red blood cells. If you are anemic you will most likely feel tired and sluggish, so much so that rest does not make you feel better.

➤ **Unusual stomach or gas pain**

➤ **Unexplained weight loss**

➤ **Fatigue**

➤ **Vomiting**

If you experience any of these symptoms, it is important to see your doctor to ensure proper diagnosis and treatment. Early diagnosis and treatment can save your life.

Risk Factors

Everyone is at risk for colorectal cancer. One out of every 50 people, or two percent of the U.S. population, will get colorectal cancer. The majority of people who develop colorectal cancer have no known risk factors; and although the exact cause of colorectal cancer is not known, there are some factors that increase a person's risk of developing the disease.

These include:

▷ **Age.** The risk of developing colorectal cancer increases as we age. The disease is more common in people over 50, and the chance of getting colorectal cancer increases with each decade. However, colorectal cancer has also been known to develop in younger people.

▷ **Gender.** Women have a higher risk for colon cancer, while men are more likely to develop rectal cancer.

▷ **Polyps.** Polyps are non-cancerous growths on the inner wall of the colon or rectum. While they are fairly common in people over 50, one type of polyp, referred to as an adenoma, increases the risk of developing colorectal cancer. Adenomas are non-cancerous polyps that are considered precursors, or the first step, toward colon and rectal cancer.

▷ **Personal history.** Research shows that women who have a history of ovarian, uterine, or breast cancer have a somewhat increased risk of developing colorectal cancer. Also, a person who has already had colorectal cancer may develop the disease a second time. In addition, people who have chronic inflammatory conditions of the colon, such as ulcerative colitis or Crohn's disease, are also at a higher risk of developing colorectal cancer.

▷ **Family history.** Parents, siblings, and children of a person who has had colorectal cancer are somewhat more likely to develop colorectal cancer themselves. If many family members have had colorectal cancer, the risk increases even more. A family history of familial polyposis, adenomous polyps, or hereditary polyp syndrome also increases the risk.

▷ **Diet.** A diet high in fat and calories and low in fiber may be linked to a greater risk of developing colorectal cancer.

> **Lifestyle factors.** You may be at increased risk for developing colorectal cancer if you drink alcohol, smoke, don't get enough exercise, and if you are overweight.

> **Diabetes.** People with diabetes have a thirty to forty percent increased risk of developing colon cancer.

Nutrition for Colon Cancer

A high-fat, high caloric diet appears to be a risk factor for colon cancer. Americans consume entirely too much fat and not nearly enough fiber, nature's colon cleanser.

The following advice may help you prevent colon cancer:

☆ Whole-grain breads are low in fat and high in fiber and complex carbohydrates. Select whole-grain breads for sandwiches and as additions to meals. Avoid rich bakery foods such as donuts, sweet rolls, and muffins. These foods can contain more than fifty percent fat calories. If you crave a sweet snack, try angel food cake or gingersnap cookies to satisfy your sweet tooth without adding fat to your diet.

☆ Granola cereals may have high-fat oils and extra sugars. Instant cereals with cream may also have high-fat oils or butterfat. Always read the label on cereal before you buy.

☆ Avoid fried snacks such as potato chips and tortilla chips. Try the low-fat or baked versions.

☆ Eat at least nine to thirteen servings of vegetables and fruits a day. Fruits and vegetables are naturally low in fat.

☆ Margarine, butter, mayonnaise, and sour cream add fat to vegetables and fruits. Use herbs and yogurt as seasonings instead.

★ Select low-fat, lean cuts of meat. Baking, broiling, and roasting are the healthiest ways to prepare meat. Lean cuts can be pan-broiled or stir-fried. Use either a nonstick pan or nonstick spray coating. Trim outside fat before cooking. Trim any inside fat before eating. Use herbs, spices, fresh vegetables, and nonfat marinades to season meat. Avoid high-fat sauces and gravies.

★ Chicken breasts are a good choice because they are low in fat. Baking, broiling, and roasting are the healthiest ways to prepare poultry. Skinless poultry can be pan-broiled or stir-fried. Use either a nonstick pan or nonstick spray coating. Remove skin and visible fat before cooking. Choose low-fat breast cuts. Use domestic goose and duck only once in a while because both are high in fat.

★ Most seafood is low in saturated fat. Poaching, steaming, baking, and broiling are the healthiest ways to prepare fish. Fresh fish should have firm, springy flesh; a clear color; a moist look; and a clean smell. If good-quality fresh fish isn't available, buy frozen fish. Omega-3 fatty acids, found in some fatty fish such as salmon and cold water trout, may help lower the risk of heart disease in some people.

★ Dry beans, peas, and lentils offer protein and fiber without the cholesterol and fat that meats have. Once in a while, try substituting beans for meat in a favorite recipe, for example, in lasagna or chili.

★ Choose skim milk or buttermilk. Substitute evaporated skim milk for cream in recipes for soups and sauces.

★ Try low-fat cheeses. Skim ricotta can replace cream cheese on a bagel or in a vegetable dip. Use part-skim mozzarella instead of cheddar cheese in recipes. Try low-fat natural or cheddar cheeses. Use one percent cottage cheese for salads and cooking. Eat string cheese as a low-fat, high-calcium snack.

⭐ Plain nonfat yogurt can replace sour cream in many recipes. Try frozen nonfat or low-fat yogurt for dessert.

⭐ Skim sherbet is an alternative to ice cream. Soft-serve and regular ice creams are lower in fat than premium styles.

✱ **Choosing Protein and Dairy Products**

As with produce, when choosing protein and dairy products we recommend they be all-natural and hormone free.

Being overweight is a risk factor in many chronic diseases. Inactivity has definitely been linked to colon cancer. Regular exercise encourages better digestion and elimination.

Adhering to the guidelines provided above will help you avoid not only colon cancer but also many other chronic disorders and diseases that are affected by diet and lifestyle.

---

*For healthy elimination try **Ultimate Living Fiber Cleanse. Fiber Cleanse** is also an excellent colon detoxifier.*

Leukemia

Leukemia is a disorder affecting the production of white blood cells, causing them to reproduce uncontrollably, crowding out existing healthy cells.

These abnormal white cells proliferate in the bone marrow, often with immature, nonfunctioning blast cells, and spill over into the bloodstream. Leukemia cells infiltrate all the major organs of the body, sometimes causing these organs to malfunction or fail. The kidneys may become impaired. The liver and spleen may become enlarged.

The cause of leukemia in most circumstances is not known. Some cases appear to be genetic in origin. Others may be related to exposure to toxins, chemicals, drugs, or radiation. Modern lifestyle factors, such as exposure to radiation, benzene, and environmental pollutants, are thought to play a major role in the rising incidence. More recent research is looking at the effect of diet and nutrition.

Many complementary therapies–from vitamins and herbal therapies to massage and acupuncture–seem to work well for persons with blood-related cancers, helping to relieve the side effects of the radiation and chemotherapy involved in the standard medical treatments.

Leukemia is more common in young children and older people than in the general adult population.

Symptoms

Symptoms of leukemia include:

▶ *Unexplained fevers*

▶ *Frequent infections*

▶ *Night sweats*

▶ *Feeling tired or washed out*

▶ *Weight loss*

▶ *Bleeding or bruising easily*

Leukemia cells in certain parts of the body may cause the following symptoms:

- Headache
- Confusion
- Balance problems
- Blurry vision
- Painful swellings in the neck, under the arms, or in the groin
- Nausea or vomiting
- Abdominal pain
- Testicular pain or swelling
- Pain in the bones or joint
- Weakness or loss of muscle control
- Seizures

The symptoms of leukemia are nonspecific and are common to a number of diseases and conditions. Your physician is able to distinguish leukemia from the other conditions that cause similar symptoms.

Nutrition for Leukemia

Nutrition essential for a leukemia patient includes protein, carbohydrates, fat, water, vitamins, and minerals.

> *Ultimate Living Ionic Trace Minerals* are 26 times more concentrated than colloidal minerals. Our *Ionic Trace Minerals* will replace minerals missing from the typical diet providing over fifty minerals in nature's perfect balance.

Protein

The body uses protein to promote growth, repair tissue, and maintain the lining of the gastrointestinal tract, skin, blood cells, and immune system. Children with leukemia who do not get enough protein may be slow to recover from illness and are especially vulnerable to infection.

After a patient undergoes treatment, he or she will need extra protein to heal tissues and to help prevent infection.

Protein is essential for a child's growth and development. In a child with leukemia, this need escalates dramatically. A child with leukemia may need as much as fifty percent more protein than a healthy child.

Vitamins and Minerals

Everyone needs vitamins and minerals, but cancer patients, particularly children, need many more of these nutrients to help with healing and, in the case of children, with proper growth and development. Speak to your health care provider about taking supplements, particularly if side effects from treatment are causing nausea and limiting dietary intake.

Carbohydrates and Fats

Carbohydrates and fats provide the body with the calories it needs for fuel. Energy can be in short supply when a person is undergoing cancer treatment.

Children being treated for cancer need even more calories for energy and healing. They may require as much as twenty percent more caloric intake than a healthy child.

Water

Water and fluids are essential to avoid dehydration, which produces undue stress on the system. Nausea and vomiting can very quickly produce dehydration.

To test for dehydration, pinch the skin over the breastbone. It should return to normal very quickly. If not, dehydration is indicated. More serious symptoms include dryness in the lining of the mouth, darker color of the urine, listlessness, and dizziness.

Recent News

Rochester, N.Y., Feb. 23, 2005 (United Press International): Scientists at the University of Rochester, N.Y., say a plant known as feverfew is the source of an agent that kills human leukemia stem cells.

A compound found in the daisy-plant, also known as bachelor's button, kills the cells as does no other single therapy, said a team from the university's James Wilmot Cancer Center.

The team said they collaborated with University of Kentucky chemists who identified a water-soluble molecule that has the same properties as parthenolide, a main component of the plant. According to the researchers, it will take months before a useable pharmaceutical compound can be made.

The National Cancer Institute has accepted the discovery into its rapid access program, which aims to move experimental drugs from the laboratory to human clinical trials as quickly as possible.

Lung Cancer

Lung cancer occurs when cells in the lung start to grow rapidly in an uncontrolled manner. Lung cancer can start anywhere in the lungs and affect any part of the respiratory system. It is the leading cause of cancer deaths in both men and women.

> **Fact:** *Smoking is responsible for eighty-seven percent of all lung cancer cases and thirty percent of all deaths from cancer.*

While several causes of lung cancer have been identified, tobacco smoke is estimated to cause the vast majority of lung cancers. Harmful substances, called carcinogens, in tobacco smoke damage the cells in the lungs. Exposure to other harmful substances, such as arsenic, asbestos, radioactive dust, and radon, can also increase the risk for lung cancer.

There are two main types of lung cancer: non–small cell lung cancer and small cell lung cancer. Non-small cell lung cancer is more common than small cell lung cancer. Over eighty percent of all lung cancers are non-small cell cancer. It generally grows and spreads more slowly than small cell lung cancer. Small cell lung cancer is less common than non-small cell lung cancer. About twenty percent of lung cancers are small cell. This type of cancer grows very rapidly, and in over eighty percent of cases it has already spread to other organs in the body by the time it is diagnosed. Small cell lung cancer is more strongly linked to smoking.

Symptoms

In the early stages of lung cancer, you may not have any symptoms. As a result, only about fifteen percent of lung cancers are diagnosed in the early stages when treatment is most effective.

Symptoms of more advanced lung cancer may include the following:

- A new cough or a cough that does not go away. Smokers who have a chronic cough from smoking may have a change in the frequency or severity of their cough.

- Chest, shoulder, or back pain that doesn't go away and often is made worse by deep breathing. About five percent of lung cancers spread to the chest wall, which can cause persistent chest pain.

- New wheezing.

- Shortness of breath.

- Hoarseness.

- Coughing up blood or bloody mucus.

- Swelling in the neck and face.

- Difficulty swallowing.

- Weight loss and loss of appetite.

- Increasing fatigue and weakness.

- Recurring respiratory infections such as pneumonia.

- Clubbing of the fingers and toes. The nails appear to bulge out more than normal.

Smoking

Smoking is the single biggest cause of lung cancer. If you smoke, STOP! The more you smoke, the more likely you are to get lung cancer, but it is the length of time you have been a smoker that is most important.

Filtered and low tar cigarettes might reduce risk slightly, but most smokers cancel this out by taking more and deeper puffs or by smoking more cigarettes.

As soon as you stop smoking, your risk of lung cancer starts to go down.

Fifteen years after you have stopped smoking, your risk of getting lung cancer is reduced to that of a non-smoker.

Passive smoking (breathing other people's cigarette smoke) does increase the risk of lung cancer, but the risk is still much less than if you smoke yourself.

Nutrition and Lung Cancer

Patients with lung cancer often have a loss of appetite and/or weight loss. These are caused by multiple factors. The tumor releases chemicals, which can cause both the weight loss and lack of appetite. Also, feeling ill, tired, or depressed can lead to both symptoms.

Treatments can also cause loss of appetite, nausea/vomiting, and fatigue, which can all lead to weight loss and poor nutrition. Radiation to the chest can cause esophagitis (inflammation and pain of the esophagus), leading to an inability to swallow liquids and/or solids until the esophagus heals.

Weight loss in lung cancer patients can be serious. Poor nutrition can lead to loss of protein in the body, which can cause muscle wasting, weakness, swelling, or fluid retention and leave you more susceptible to infection.

There are ways to manage the symptoms and boost the appetite:

- Eat small, frequent meals.
- Increase your protein intake. Examples of foods rich in protein include cheese, meat, eggs, and dairy products.

- Supplement your diet with good quality protein shakes.

> **Ultimate Living Green Miracle** added to a protein shake will provide you with extra nutrients and valuable nutrition as well as your daily requirement of fruits and vegetables.

- Drink plenty of fluids and limit caffeine consumption.

- If you are nauseated from treatment, avoid the kitchen while food is being prepared so the smells will not bother you.

- Eat, eat, eat–wasting or uncontrolled weight loss is a major problem for lung cancer patients.

With the rise in pollution levels and ozone, lung cancer has become more common in individuals who do not smoke, but smoking remains far and away the major cause of lung cancer. Stopping today puts you on a road to diminishing risk.

As with any disease, a healthy lifestyle with good nutrition, exercise, and lack of stress will help your immune system fight cancer. The lungs appear to be one of the cancer sites that respond positively to the consumption of fruits and vegetables. In fact, it is thought that persons who have maintained a healthy diet throughout their lives, including sufficient quantities of vegetables and fruits, experience better survival rates when diagnosed with lung cancer.

Overcoming Side Effects of Cancer Treatment

In the course of your treatment, you may feel mildly ill, be overcome by nausea, or have bouts of vomiting. These things can occur before, during, right after, and days after you receive your chemotherapy. They can be caused by the cancer itself or by its treatment.

The following are some tips to help you manage nausea and vomiting:

- Breathing through your nose deeply and slowly can help with nausea.

- Eat smaller meals throughout the day.

- Avoid sweet, fried, or fatty foods.

- If cooking odors offend you, stay away from the kitchen while food is being prepared. If you are making your own meals, eat food at room temperature or cold until your nausea subsides.

- If you are ill in the mornings, try a little dry toast or crackers before arising (be careful if you have mouth sores or dry mouth).

- Try apple or grape juice or light-color sodas, such as ginger ale.

- Try ginger tea, fresh ginger, and pickled and candied ginger. Ginger is an ancient remedy for sour stomach. Sometimes just sniffing a cut surface of fresh ginger can help with mild nausea.

- Making certain you are getting enough fluids can help minimize nausea. Aim for six to eight glasses of fluids a day. Avoid eating large meals, spicy foods, or acidic foods (such as tomatoes, lemons, and oranges). Stick with bland foods such as bananas, rice, unsweetened applesauce, toast, and potatoes (not fried).

- Nausea or queasiness from anxiety can be improved with both mindful measures and medications. Visualization and meditation can be particularly helpful. Acupuncture can also be quite effective at relieving nausea.

- Some people claim that the "sea band" worn on boats or airplanes can help ease nausea. These are available at most larger drug stores. Make sure you read the directions carefully so that you know where the band should go.

> ***Ultimate Living Aloe-Papaya Drink*** *is a great way to settle your stomach.*

Fatigue and Depression

Fatigue is the most common side effect of cancer treatment. But proper nutrition, vitamin and mineral supplements, medications, lifestyle changes, and emotional support can help give you the energy you need to enjoy your life.

Here are some tips to help you enjoy each day, even during treatment!

▷ **Plan Your Day**

- Take note of the times of day when you feel your best.

- Plan your activities, rest periods, and household tasks according to your energy level.

- Get plenty of rest, and balance your activities. Don't overdo.

- Don't be afraid to ask for help with chores and errands. Your family and friends want to help.

▷ **Eat Well**

- Eat lots of fruits, vegetables, whole grains, and protein to fuel your body.

> *Ultimate Living Green Miracle,* a live food, will provide all the nutrients required to help rebuild your immune system.

- Talk to your doctor about vitamins and nutritional supplements that might help.

- Use healthful, easy-to-prepare foods whenever possible.

- Shop for groceries when the supermarket is not busy.

- When you feel well, do some cooking and freeze individual portions.

▷ **Do things you enjoy**

- Find a park or garden where you can restore mental energy.

- Get regular exercise. Walk at a pace that doesn't make you overly tired.

- Talk with a trusted friend, family member, or clergy about what you're going through.

- Find a cancer support group. Talking with others facing similar problems can be very rewarding.

- Read spiritually uplifting books.

Pain Management

Having cancer should not mean living with pain. Many people with cancer do not have pain. Cancer pain can almost always be relieved if you work closely with your health care professionals to set up a treatment plan for the pain. Learn about different methods of controlling pain, including medications and other techniques such as relaxation and biofeedback. It is important to develop and adopt a pain management plan that keeps you on top of the pain. Once pain has taken hold, it is more difficult to control.

Support

If you are going through cancer and cancer treatment, it can be very consoling and helpful to talk with people who are having or have had similar experiences. Support groups are a good place to meet with fellow cancer patients and a wonderful resource for information. Often there are patients who have had experiences that they can share that may help you down the road. Perhaps they have experienced or researched a treatment that you are considering.

Your local American Cancer Society chapter can provide you with lists of cancer support groups and those specific to your needs. Your hospital or health care provider should also be able to provide you with contacts and groups.

Chapter Nine

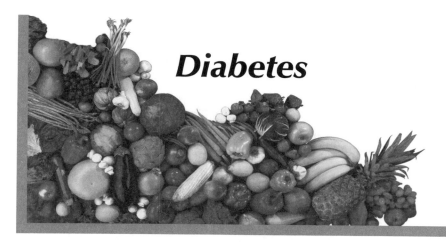

Diabetes

T he number of people diagnosed with diabetes is growing in epidemic proportions in this country. A debilitating disease, diabetes leads to other serious chronic conditions such as heart disease, kidney failure, and digestive disorders as well as blindness and amputations.

Diabetes is a serious chronic condition where the body either does not make or does not properly use insulin. The result is that sugar builds up in the bloodstream rather being processed by the cells. Subsequently, the body cannot produce the energy it needs from food ingested. Diabetes affects about twenty million people in the United States and 300 million people worldwide.

There are several types of diabetes. The most common are types 1 and 2. Causes of diabetes include heredity, immune system dysfunction, and viruses. There are also contributing factors such as obesity, lack of exercise, and poor nutrition. The consumption of high glycemic (sugar), high-fat, and nutrient-deficient foods puts you at risk for diabetes.

Type 1 Diabetes

In type 1 or insulin-dependent diabetes, also known as juvenile diabetes, the body produces little or no insulin, meaning that sugar cannot enter

161

cells to be used for energy and the blood sugar levels remain high. With this type, diabetics must take insulin. Although type 1 is usually diagnosed in children, its symptoms can appear suddenly and at any age. Type 1 diabetes accounts for about ten percent of all diabetes.

Symptoms of type 1 diabetes include the following:

- Increased hunger
- Increased thirst
- Increased urination
- Sudden weight loss
- Fatigue

The pancreas contains beta cells which make insulin, a hormone that helps cells absorb sugar. In type 1 diabetes, the immune system malfunctions, and cells that normally protect you from germs attack and kill your beta cells in error. Without beta cells, no insulin is produced, and sugar builds up in the blood. The result is diabetes.

The key to a healthy and long life with Type 1 diabetes is the monitoring of blood sugar levels and endeavoring to keep them within a target range. This can be achieved through consistent and careful meal planning, exercise, and the administration of insulin. There are very accurate glucose monitoring kits on the market. Your endocrinologist will advise you on how often you need to test depending on the nature and severity of your diabetes.

Type 2 Diabetes

Type 2 diabetes, or adult-onset diabetes, used to be referred to as non-insulin diabetes. Although usually found in older people, recently the number of young people with this type has been on the rise.

Type 2 is by far the more common of the two diabetic conditions. Here the body is either not producing enough insulin or the cells are ignoring the insulin. As you have learned, insulin is critical in cellular energy. It is the hormone that enables the body to use sugar. Sugar is the basic fuel for the cells in the body, and insulin takes the sugar from the bloodstream into the cells. When glucose is allowed to build up in the blood rather than being used in the cells, it causes two problems: cells may become starved for energy, and, over time, high blood sugar levels can hurt your eyes, kidneys, nerves, or heart.

In people with type 2 diabetes, glucose builds up, but with proper treatment the levels return to normal. This, however, does not mean you are cured, only that you are controlling your diabetes. It is important to be very consistent. Meal planning, exercise, and weight loss are very helpful. There are new medications that can be taken orally to control this type of diabetes. Rarely do type 2 patients need to take insulin injections although they are required if glucose levels can be controlled by no other means.

Symptoms of type 2 diabetes include:

- Increased hunger, thirst, urination
- Blurred vision
- Fatigue
- Numbness or tingling in the hands and feet
- Impotence
- Dry, itchy skin
- Slow healing cuts or sores
- Frequent infections

Prediabetes

Prediabetes, also called impaired glucose tolerance (IGT), is a precursor condition to type 2 diabetes. It is characterized by higher than normal blood glucose levels and insulin resistance. The American Diabetes Association and National Institutes of Health estimate that over forty million Americans have prediabetes, and only a fraction of these have been diagnosed with the condition. The risk factors for prediabetes are the same as those for type 2 diabetes.

Gestational Diabetes

Gestational diabetes, or diabetes that occurs in pregnancy and is resolved after giving birth, occurs in approximately three to eight of every 100 pregnancies in America.

Risk factors for developing gestational diabetes include these:

- A family history of diabetes
- Being overweight
- Having prediabetes
- Having given birth previously to a child weighing nine pounds or more

In addition, the same populations at risk for type 2 diabetes–Hispanic Americans, African Americans, Pacific Islanders, and Asian Americans– are also at greater risk for gestational diabetes.

Hypoglycemia

While diabetes is a disease where blood sugar is too high, hypoglycemia is a condition in which the blood sugar is too low. Left untreated, hypoglycemia can escalate into diabetes.

Symptoms of hypoglycemia are:

- Feeling shaky or weak
- Sweating
- Dizziness
- Overwhelming fatigue
- Rapid heartbeat
- Numbness or tingling in the mouth or lips
- Hunger

Symptoms that indicate an escalating problem are:

- Crying
- Irritability or anger
- Drowsiness
- Mental confusion and/or difficulty thinking
- Poor coordination
- Blurred vision and/or headaches
- Slurred Speech

Hypoglycemia is caused by several physiological reasons. Everyday causes may include taking too much insulin if you are diabetic, eating at the wrong time or skipping meals, exercising too much without enough food, and, most commonly, improper nutrition.

For diabetics, experiencing a hypoglycemic or low blood sugar episode can be scary—both for the diabetic and for others who may be present. Prompt and appropriate treatment of lows is critical to avoiding an emergency situation, so make sure you're always prepared with a fast-acting carbohydrate source, blood testing supplies, and medical identification. And share the information with friends, family, and co-workers so that they know how to help should you be unable to treat yourself.

If you experience any symptoms of low blood sugar levels, including sweating, lightheadedness, shakiness, confusion, anxiety, unexplained anger, hunger, and fatigue, act quickly to bring your blood sugars back to safe levels.

Blood sugar imbalances are quite common. The symptoms of hypoglycemia and diabetes are a clear indication that the body is not processing or metabolizing glucose properly. Signs that this is the case are fatigue, depression, stress, and obesity. Many people discount these indications and attribute them to other reasons. It is important to listen to your body. If you have a combination of these symptoms, glucose imbalance might be your problem; and certainly, if you suspect diabetes, you should see your physician immediately.

Ketones

If for any reason your body can't use glucose, it has an alternative–fat. To use fat as a fuel, your body first has to break it down into small pieces; these small pieces are called ketones. For people with type 1 diabetes and for some with type 2, ketones can be a problem. Raised levels can lead to diabetic ketoacidosis and possibly a trip to the emergency room.

Chapter Nine: Diabetes

Everyone at some point uses ketones as fuel. For example, someone who doesn't eat for a while will burn ketones, so you may have a small amount of ketones in your blood first thing in the morning. Energetic exercise can also make ketone levels rise when all the glucose has been used. In both cases, ketone levels rise, but blood glucose levels do not.

When you have diabetes, rising blood glucose and rising blood ketones can go together. Insulin is needed to move glucose from your blood into your muscles and brain so they can use it as fuel. When you don't have enough insulin in your blood, your body will begin to turn fat into ketones to use as fuel instead. This is not good news for people with diabetes. Without insulin your body goes on making ketones, and your levels can get dangerously high.

Diabetic ketoacidosis may lead to the initial diagnosis of type 1 diabetes as it is often the first symptom that causes the person to come to medical attention. People with type 2 diabetes usually develop ketoacidosis only under conditions of severe stress.

There are three times when you may be particularly at risk from raised ketone levels:

- If your diabetes has recently been diagnosed or your medication has been changed.

- If you don't monitor your blood glucose regularly

- If you are ill

More glucose is produced as a result of the body's defense mechanism for fighting illness. You can make glucose from your own body stores. Normally extra insulin would then be produced to move this glucose from your blood into your muscles. But if you don't have enough insulin to meet the demand, your body turns to fat, its other source of fuel, to make energy, and the by-products of that are ketones.

High levels of ketones are harmful, so, as soon as they start to rise, your body tries to get rid of them in your urine. Consequently, early signs of rising ketones are a need to urinate more often and feeling thirsty. (Remember, your blood glucose levels will also be high, and this will also be causing you to pass water more frequently and to feel thirsty.)

If your ketone levels continue to rise, they act like a poison. You may feel sick and find it difficult to keep liquids down, making you even more dehydrated. Your skin may become dry and your eyesight blurred, and you may find you are breathing faster. Ketones can be smelled on your breath. Your breath will have a distinctly sweet and sickly smell.

Sometimes it is difficult to know at first if a raised blood glucose reading is just inaccurate or something serious. But the earlier you detect rising blood ketones, the easier it may be for you and your physician to bring them back down.

There are two ways of detecting rising ketones:

- Urine testing
- Blood testing

Diabetic Disorders

If left uncontrolled, diabetes can lead to other serious health problems.

These include:

> **Neuropathy.** Nerve damage is among the most common complications related to diabetes and can extend to all areas of the body.

> **Heart disease.** With diabetes comes an increased risk of heart attack.

> **Poor eye health, blindness.** Diabetics face a higher risk of diabetic retinopathy which can lead to blindness. Diabetics need to have their eyes checked frequently by a qualified health care professional.

> **Kidney disease.** Damaged kidneys prevent the body from properly eliminating waste products.

> **Skin problems.** The American Diabetes Association (ADA) estimates that as many as one-third of all diabetics will have a skin disorder linked to the disease. Skin conditions very often are the first symptoms of the disease.

> **Oral health.** Diabetics face a higher risk of gum disease.

> **Foot problems.** Usually a result of neuropathy, foot problems are a result of nerve problems progressing into the lower extremities. Circulation complications that stem from diabetes can also lead to foot problems. It is important that diabetics maintain proper foot care, paying particular attention to recurring nail fungus which, if left untreated, can lead to serious skin and bone infections, and even tissue death resulting in the necessity for amputation.

Diabetes and Lifestyle

Most cases of type 2, the most common form of diabetes, can be prevented by moderate exercise and a healthy diet. Studies indicate that such lifestyle changes could halt over ninety percent of type 2 diabetes cases and that the changes could reduce the risk of getting the disease by some fifty-eight percent even among those already showing symptoms.

Researchers definitely believe that diabetes is a lifestyle disease. They have concluded that a vast number of occurrences of the disease could be prevented by being active, eating right, not drinking alcohol, not smoking, and by avoiding being overweight.

Being overweight is the single strongest predictor of diabetes. Over sixty percent of all cases can be attributed to weight problems. Overweight women can, however, cut their risk by almost twenty-five percent simply by walking regularly and selecting foods high in fiber but low in partially hydrogenated oils (French fries, commercially baked goods).

The benefits of exercise seem to climb with the level of physical activity. People who exercise seven or more hours a week have a thirty percent lower risk of diabetes than do those who exercise only one hour per week. A good, healthy diet offers similar benefits.

The good news is that these lifestyle changes are easy–things all of us can do.

Nutrition and Diabetes

The ADA recommends that people with diabetes follow this type of dietary plan:

- Eat on a schedule

- Eat nutrition-based foods rather than "empty" calories

- Regularly monitor blood sugar levels and adjust immediately when needed

- Adopt a steady regimen of exercise

- Eat snacks around the same time each day to keep sugar levels stable

Additional suggestions are:

- Plan your meals so that you eat healthy food, not just whatever is easiest

- Think before you eat instead of raiding the refrigerator every time you feel hungry

- Use a smaller plate so that you can't heap on much more than you really want or need

- Chew slowly and completely, savoring every mouthful, instead of packing in as much as you can as quickly as you can

For diabetics, eating healthy means you should avoid foods containing sugary sweets and large amounts of carbohydrates. Both of these can cause blood sugar levels to rise to extreme levels.

Eating quality, organic vegetables is very helpful. Green vegetables supply slow-acting (low stress) carbohydrates. They are nutrition-rich and have virtually no effect on sugar levels. The consumption of high starch foods, particularly French fries as well as highly refined foods such as pastas and some breads, may be one of the main reasons this country is facing diabetes at epidemic levels. The average American diet is the perfect springboard for diabetes. Many people in the United States literally live on fast foods.

Maintaining a healthy diet is important for everyone, but it is especially important for people with diabetes.

Following the right meal plan can make all the difference to persons struggling to keep their blood sugar under control. Diet is a vital component in your overall diabetes control program. Your health providers can assist you in developing a personal meal plan to help you attain and maintain proper blood sugar and blood fat (cholesterol and triglyceride) levels.

If you have non-insulin dependent diabetes, sticking to your meal plan helps you achieve and maintain your correct weight and balances the foods you eat with the insulin your body produces. If you have insulin dependent diabetes, you must stick to your meal plan to insure a balance between injected insulin and the foods you eat.

Carb Counting

Carbohydrates provide fuel for the body in the form of glucose. There are two types of carbohydrates, simple and complex. Simple carbohydrates are sugars; they are found in refined sugar and in fruits. Complex carbohydrates are the starches; they are found in beans, nuts, vegetables, and whole grains. Complex carbohydrates are considered very healthy, mostly because they are digested by the body slowly and provide a steady source of energy. Carbohydrates have the most immediate effect on your blood glucose since they are broken down into sugar early during digestion. It is important to eat the suggested amount of carbohydrates at each meal along with some protein and fat.

Carbohydrates are mainly found in three food groups: fruit; milk and yogurt; and bread, cereal, rice, pasta, and starchy vegetables. Counting grams of carbohydrate and evenly distributing them at meals will help you control your blood glucose. Carbohydrate counting is a method of meal planning that is a simple way to keep track of the amount of total carbohydrates you eat each day.

A registered dietitian will help you figure out a carbohydrate counting plan that meets your specific needs. For adults, a typical plan generally includes three to four carbohydrate choices at each meal and one to two carbohydrate choices as snacks. With carbohydrate counting, you can pick almost any food product off the shelf, read the label, and use the information about grams of carbohydrate to fit the food into your meal plan.

Carbohydrate counting may not be for everyone, and the traditional method of following food exchange lists may be used instead.

Exchange Lists

Your dietitian may use exchange lists to help you plan meals and snacks. Exchange lists are groups of foods that contain roughly the same mix of carbohydrates, protein, fat, and calories. There are six exchange lists:

★ *Starches and breads*

★ *Meats and meat substitutes*

★ *Vegetables*

★ *Fruits*

★ *Milk*

★ *Fats*

You need foods from all six lists for complete nutrition. Foods on the exchange lists are familiar, everyday items you can buy at the supermarket. The exchange lists are the basis of a meal planning system designed by a committee of the American Diabetes Association and the American Dietetic Association. While designed primarily for people with diabetes and others who must follow special diets, the exchange lists are based on principles of good nutrition that apply to everyone.

Glycemic Index

Some researchers think that a low-glycemic index diet may be the way to go. Even foods with the same carbohydrate content can trigger a wide difference in blood sugar levels–as much as fivefold. Researchers say it depends on the food's glycemic index, a number that indicates how much and how quickly blood sugar increases after consuming a carbohydrate-containing food. Although important, the numbers can also be confusing because the glycemic index of some foods may surprise you. As a general rule, the same low-fat, high-fiber foods that are often recommended for helping to manage weight and prevent diabetes and other health problems such as fruits, vegetables, whole grains, and legumes also have low glycemic indexes. Starchy and processed foods such as potatoes, breads, and cereals usually have a high glycemic index.

There are some exceptions.

- For instance, a bowl of All-Bran cereal has a glycemic index of 54 while a serving of spaghetti rates at 41, meaning the high-fiber cereal spikes blood glucose more quickly and drastically.

- A handful of raisins is 64, more than a serving of popcorn at 55.

- White rice (56) has nearly twice the glycemic index of a glass of apple juice

- An orange (43) has almost half the index of watermelon (72).

The American Journal of Clinical Nutrition lists any food under 55 as a low-glycemic food and any food more than 70 as high glycemic. The use of diets with a low glycemic index in the treatment of diabetes remains controversial and continues to be researched.

The Basics

Although foods contain many nutrients, it is easiest to categorize them into three groups:

- **Carbohydrate foods** include bread, potatoes, rice, crackers, cookies, sugar, fruit, vegetables, and pasta. When digested, carbohydrates provide fuel for energy.

▷ **Protein foods** include meat, poultry, fish, eggs, cheese, dried beans, and legumes. When digested, protein is used to build and repair your body. Some protein may also be used as fuel for energy.

▷ **Fat foods** include butter, margarine, cooking oil, cream, bacon, and nuts. When digested, fats are stored as fat cells or later used as fuel for energy.

Your meal plan should include carbohydrates, proteins, and fats in amounts that will promote good diabetes control while providing adequate fuel for energy and building and repairing your body. Your health provider can assist with your plan. Further, the American Diabetes Association offers dietary suggestions.

Reduce Sugar

Don't eat sugar and avoid honey, syrup, jam, jelly, candy, sweet rolls, regular gelatin, cake with icing, and pie. Instead of fruit canned in syrup, choose fresh fruit or fruit canned in natural juice or water. Do not drink colas. One twelve-ounce can of regular cola contains nine teaspoons of sugar!

Increase Fiber

Fiber, also known as roughage, is the part of plant food your body cannot digest. Fiber relieves constipation, lowers blood cholesterol levels, and slows down the rate of carbohydrate digestion, reducing carbohydrate-induced elevations of blood sugar.

Increase your intake of fiber by:

● switching to whole-grain breads, cereals, and crackers.

- eating more vegetables—raw and cooked. Instead of fruit juice, eat fresh, whole fruit.

- consuming high-fiber foods such as bran, barley, bulgur; brown and wild rice, and dried beans, peas, and lentils.

Reduce Sodium

Don't add salt in cooking, and try not to put salt on your food at the table. Cut down on high-salt foods such as canned soups, ham, sauerkraut, hot dogs, and pickles. Food that tastes salty probably is salty. Eat fewer convenience foods and try to avoid fast-food restaurants.

Fast foods and convenience foods are often loaded with sodium.

Eat Less Fat

Cut down on meat. Eat more fish and poultry instead. When you do eat red meat, choose the leanest cuts. Roast, bake, or broil instead of frying. Trim the fat off meat and the skin off poultry and avoid adding fat in cooking. Beware of sauces and gravies; they often contain lots of fat. Eliminate or cut down on high-fat foods such as cold cuts, bacon, sausage, hot dogs, butter, margarine, nuts, salad dressings, lard, and shortening.

Delicious low-fat versions of ice cream, cheese, sour cream, and cream are increasingly available in grocery stores. Drink skim or low-fat milk instead of whole milk.

Cinnamon

> *A dash of cinnamon could significantly lower your cholesterol, triglycerides, and blood sugar.*

According to researchers at the USDA's Beltsville Human Nutrition Research Center in Maryland, when thirty women and men with type 2 diabetes added a sprinkle of cinnamon to their meals, blood sugar and heart-damaging blood fats (total cholesterol and triglycerides) fell twelve to thirty percent in just forty days.

Recommendations are for small amounts: about 1/6 teaspoon at breakfast, lunch, and dinner, for a daily total of about 1/2 teaspoon. Since cinnamon may reduce your need for diabetes or cholesterol medication, ask your doctor if you need to adjust your dose.

Stress management

Stress particularly exacerbates diabetic conditions for several reasons. Under stress, the body's defense mechanism gears up for the "fight or flight" situation. Hormonal levels shoot up and release extra sugar to provide energy. A diabetic already has problems in using the sugar in the blood. With extra sugar in the blood, the condition worsens. Under stress, many people fail to exercise, forget to take medicines, and drink or smoke more (if they have the habit) in an attempt to escape stress.

The trick is to combat stress. Relaxation techniques such as meditation, imagery, and exercise can help.

Avoiding smoking and drinking

Smoking is addictive and increases your chance of cancer and heart diseases. Smoking also narrows the peripheral blood vessels and makes it difficult for wounds on the hands and legs to heal quickly. Drinking affects your liver. These are complications a diabetic can do without.

Exercise

If you are a diabetic, you have to keep your weight in control. You should take care of other aspects of your health, such as blood pressure and the condition of the heart, so that your sugar levels do not affect these and lead to major health problems. Exercise helps with all of these aspects.

Cardiovascular exercises are recommended. Walking is ideal. Remember to always warm up before exercising. If you have been inactive, start with a twenty minute schedule and gradually increase the duration and intensity until you are walking seven hours a week for optimum benefits.

Stretches are also beneficial. Diabetes can lead to shortening of muscles. Stretching keeps you flexible and fit. Always stretch before and after physical exertion.

If your sugar level is high in the early morning, have a workout in the evening so that blood glucose does not accumulate in the night.

There is always a chance of hypoglycemia, especially for the insulin dependent diabetes patient. If your sugar level drops as you workout, you are likely to break into a sweat and feel giddy. Keep a light snack or organic dark chocolate handy. Drink plenty of fluids to prevent dehydration.

Foot care is important. Use made-to-order diabetic footwear, especially when you are following a walking program. This keeps the pressure on the feet uniform. This also avoids corns and other foot problems that for diabetics can present real problems with slow healing and infection. If you have neuropathy, you may not feel the prick of a thorn or a mild injury to the foot. Good footwear and regular examination of the feet help prevent complications.

Supplements for Diabetics

As you have read, illness can be a real risk for diabetics so it is important that you keep your immune system strong. Many supplements, however, are off limits to persons suffering from diabetes, particularly powdered drinks that very often contain sugars.

*Ultimate Living offers a **Glucose Balance Pack** that provides excellent nutritional support for the diabetic. **Green Miracle** provides all the required servings of fruits and vegetables and is completely safe for diabetics. It contains no added sugar. **Green Miracle** contains valuable nutrition to support the immune system and to promote healing. Healing can be an especially serious problem for diabetics. The **Glucose Balance Pack** also contains our delicious **Aloe-Papaya Drink.** For centuries aloe vera has been known as the healing plant. Also in the pack are **Ultimate Living Multi-Vitamin, Ionic Trace Minerals,** and our powerful **Immune Support Formula.** The **Ultimate Living Glucose Balance Pack** is loaded with ingredients specifically designed to regulate and stabilize glucose levels. (You should always discuss any supplement program with your physician or health care provider.)*

Traditionally it was believed that the long-term complications of diabetes were inevitable. We now know that this is not necessarily true for most people. The key to a positive prognosis is control–controlling your diet, your weight, and, most importantly, your glucose levels. New and more accurate monitoring systems and the latest diabetes treatments are enabling diabetics to live longer, healthier, and more normal lives than ever before.

Chapter Ten

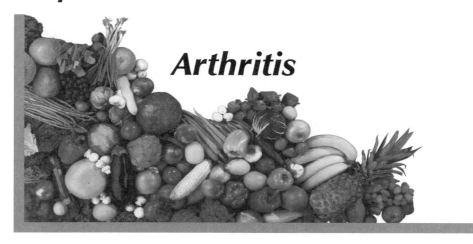

Arthritis

A rthritis or other chronic joint pain affects nearly 70 million people in America and is the number one cause of disability.

Check the shelves of your local drugstore. Listen to the preponderance of advertising. Notice the variety of new products on the market to relieve the pain of arthritis. It is clear that our country is aging. The baby-boom generation is reaching retirement, and everybody has aches and pains. Chronic pain is, in fact, a major health problem in the United States with more than seventy million Americans suffering from some form of arthritis ranging from osteoarthritis, the most common form of arthritis, to rheumatoid arthritis, the most disabling form of the disease.

The word arthritis literally means joint inflammation, but these diseases may affect not only the joints but also other parts of the body, including muscles, bones, tendons, and ligaments, as well as some internal organs. Anyone who lives long enough can almost count on developing arthritis, osteoarthritis at the very least.

There are some one hundred forms of the disease, ranging from mild forms of tendinitis and bursitis to such crippling systemic forms as rheumatoid arthritis. There are pain syndromes, such as fibromyalgia, as well as arthritis-related disorders, such as systemic lupus erythematosus, that involve every part of the body. There are forms of the disease such as gout that almost no one realizes is a form of arthritis, and there are other, more common forms of the disease such as osteoarthritis that everyone knows.

Although it is true that many older people do have arthritis, it is not simply a disease of the elderly. Some forms of arthritis affect children and young adults.

Doctors do not understand why arthritis pain varies from person to person. For instance, some people experience pain and stiffness on arising in the morning while others hurt following activity. The common factor in all these conditions is joint and musculoskeletal pain. Frequently pain is a result of inflammation of the joint lining. To compound the problem, prescription pain medicines that have seemingly worked well for arthritis pain have now been deemed dangerous, and many have been pulled from the market.

What is an arthritis sufferer to do? Let's talk about the various forms of arthritis and what can be done to relieve discomfort and help strengthen bones and connective tissue.

Osteoarthritis

Osteoarthritis, which is caused by the breakdown of cartilage, affects men and women in equal numbers; and while it is most common after the age of forty-five, it can occur at any age. Pieces of cartilage can break off and cause pain, friction, and swelling in the joints between bones. In time, cartilage may wear away entirely, allowing bones to rub together.

Osteoarthritis can affect any joint but usually affects hips, knees, hands, and spine. The symptoms of osteoarthritis include pain, stiffness, and swelling around a joint that lasts for days at a time. The most commonly affected joints are the hips, knees, feet, spine, and finger and thumb joints.

Symptoms of osteoarthritis usually come on gradually, and damage progresses slowly over time. You may have pain, especially when moving a joint, or you may hear grating sounds (friction) when damaged cartilage rubs together. Bumps and swelling may appear, especially on the extremities. Joints may feel sore and stiff, and range of motion can become limited. These changes can make it difficult, sometimes impossible, to perform simple tasks.

No one knows exactly what causes osteoarthritis, but there are a number of risk factors, including heredity, excess weight, injury, and joint damage resulting from another type of arthritis.

With the current bad news related to medications that have been successfully staving off the pain of arthritis, sufferers are in search of relief. A diagnosis of osteoarthritis, however, does not condemn you to giving up activity and suffering chronic pain. There are numerous things you can do not only to relieve the pain and stiffness but also to prevent the progression of the disease.

Exercise

As difficult as it seems when every bone in your body seems to be hurting, exercise helps reduce pain and prevents further joint damage. It can also help you maintain a healthy weight, which puts less strain on your joints. Range of motion exercises reduce stiffness and help keep your joints moving. A range of motion exercise for your shoulder, for instance, would be to move your arm in a large circle.

Strengthening exercises, such as lifting free weights, maintain or increase muscle strength. Endurance exercises, such as walking or cycling, strengthen your heart, give you energy, and help to control your weight. Moderate stretching exercises will help relieve the pain and keep the muscles and tendons around the affected joints flexible and strong. The best exercises for persons suffering with osteoarthritis are low-impact exercises such as swimming, walking, water aerobics, and stationary bicycling. Muscles and the other tissues that hold joints together weaken when they aren't moved enough. Exercise helps lessen the symptoms and can help make you feel better overall.

Hot and Cold

Although there is concern that heat can sometimes worsen an already inflamed joint, applying heat helps relax aching muscles and reduces joint pain and soreness. Heat should always be wet heat such as a hot shower or bath. Applying cold helps to lessen the swelling in a joint. Using an ice pack on the area that is sore can be very beneficial. While heat helps to reduce pain and stiffness by relaxing aching muscles and increasing circulation to the area, cold helps numb the area by constricting the blood vessels and blocking nerve impulses in the joint. Applying cold such as ice packs is the preferred treatment for inflamed joints.

In addition, there are several excellent arthritis rubs on the market that produce a warming sensation on a sore, painful joint. These can be quite soothing and effective in easing stiffness and aching.

> ***Ultimate Living Super Green Miracle Relief Gel*** *is an excellent choice. It contains emu oil; methylsulfonyl methane (MSM), an anti-inflammatory to remove pain; and arnica to relieve swelling, pain, and stiff joints in a soothing formula of aloe vera gel and menthol.*

Avoid injury

It is important to make a habit of using larger, stronger joints to carry loads. For example, carry a shoulder bag rather than one that hangs from the wrist. Avoid staying in the same position for long periods of time. Many osteoarthritis sufferers complain that sitting for hours is the worst thing they can do. A long car trip, for instance, can cause discomfort. Be sure to stop to stretch periodically. Your body will tell you the activities that exacerbate your condition. You need to listen to your body.

Lose Weight

Losing weight helps reduce the risk of osteoarthritis, and it lessens pain by reducing stress on the joints.

Relax

Relax your muscles to relieve strain on your joints. There are many ways to relax. For example, try deep breathing exercises, listening to music or relaxation tapes, meditating or praying. Another way to relax is visualization, daydreaming about a relaxing place or activity.

Fibromyalgia

Fibromyalgia is a common disease that affects from two percent to almost six percent of all people. Women are much more likely to develop fibromyalgia than men (by a ratio of four to one). Its occurrence increases with age, and it is most common in women fifty years of age or older.

If you have fibromyalgia, you may experience a number of symptoms. Common symptoms include pain and swelling in many joints or soft tissues. As a result of the pain, you may have trouble sleeping, and you may feel exhausted and weak throughout the day. Your memory may be poor, and you could have trouble concentrating. You may also feel stiff, particularly in the morning. Some people also experience numbness in joints or muscles.

In addition, you may have dry-eye, and you may develop sensitivities to heat and cold or to certain foods or medications. You may also develop allergies. Some people with fibromyalgia experience tension, migraine headaches, irritable bowel and bladder, chronic fatigue syndrome, and temperomandibular joint (TMJ) dysfunction (characterized by pain in the jaw). Depression is a common symptom in people with fibromyalgia.

Being in pain and having no energy makes it difficult to manage such normal activities as maintaining a job and housekeeping as well as recreational and other leisure pursuits. This can lead to stress and anxiety. This stress is compounded by the fact that people with fibromyalgia usually don't "look sick." It is often difficult for them to get understanding and support from family, friends, and employers, and they are sometimes even viewed as hypochondriacs.

Fibromyalgia often causes sufferers to become less active in order to avoid pain. This becomes a self-fulfilling prophecy since decreased activity causes muscles to weaken, making activity even more uncomfortable.

Researchers do not know the exact causes of fibromyalgia. For many people, this disease develops gradually without any known cause. Some doctors associate its onset to problems with the joints in the neck and lower back, motor vehicle accidents, work-related injuries, viral illnesses, surgery, infections, emotional trauma, or physical or emotional stress.

Although there is no cure for fibromyalgia, the symptoms, including pain, can be lessened by making some simple lifestyle changes. If you have fibromyalgia, you may benefit from participating in some type of **exercise** program. Because many people with fibromyalgia are not in optimum physical condition, it is important to build up the amount of exercise gradually. Exercises that may be helpful are walking, low impact aerobic programs designed for people with arthritis, water exercise programs, and the use of such exercise equipment as a stationary bike or treadmill.

Whatever exercise you choose, remember to use stretching exercises to warm up. It is not unusual to feel some soreness when you start exercising for the first time; but if your exercise program is causing an extended increase in pain, then slow down. Always listen to your body.

Applying **heat** may provide you some temporary relief of pain. Many people with fibromyalgia ease their discomfort by using a heating pad, taking a hot shower, or using a whirlpool. Heat helps to reduce pain and stiffness by relaxing aching muscles and increasing circulation to the area.

Managing your lifestyle can often be very beneficial. Do not allow yourself to become overly tired or stressed. You might keep a journal so you can begin to identify the "triggers" of your fibromyalgia. You will then know what activities to do or to forego, what foods might have an effect, etc. It is very important that you take charge of your life when you are suffering from fibromyalgia.

Rheumatoid Arthritis

Rheumatoid arthritis (RA) is an autoimmune disease that causes inflammation in the lining of the joints and/or internal organs. It is a chronic disease, affecting many joints throughout the body and resulting in damage to cartilage, bone, tendons, and ligaments. The membranes surrounding the lubricating fluid in and around the joints and often the bone surfaces are destroyed, causing stiffness, fatigue, and, in many cases, crippling pain.

Researchers believe that the inflammation of the lining of the joints is triggered by the body's immune system failing to recognize body tissue as "normal," therefore attacking it and bringing about joint damage. The damage is increased because the immune system's attack does not stop, thus resulting in the destruction of cartilage, bone, tendons, and ligaments. Such damage can lead to permanent deformity and disability. While it more commonly appears between the ages of twenty-five and fifty, RA can affect people of all ages, from toddlers to seniors. Twice as many women get RA as men.

The warning signs of RA are:

- Pain, swelling, tenderness, heat, or redness in a joint
- Joints usually affected are the hands or the feet
- Morning stiffness that lasts longer than thirty minutes
- Pain in three or more joints at the same time
- Pain in a joint all night long
- Pain in the same joints on both sides of your body
- Low energy and fatigue
- Possible fever and weight loss.

RA may start gradually or with a sudden, severe attack with flu-like symptoms, and symptoms vary from person to person. In some people, the disease will be mild with alternate periods of activity or joint inflammation (flare-ups) and inactivity (remissions). In other cases, the disease will be continuously active and appear to get worse or progress over time.

Along with painful, inflamed joints, RA can cause inflammation in other body tissues and organs. In twenty percent of cases, lumps called rheumatoid nodules develop under the skin, often over bony areas. These occur most often around the elbow but can be found elsewhere on the body and even in internal organs. Occasionally, people with RA will develop inflammation of the membranes that surround the heart and lungs or inflammation of the lung tissue itself. Inflammation of tear glands and salivary glands may cause dry eyes and dry mouth. Although it happens rarely, RA can cause inflammation of the blood vessels, thus affecting the skin, nerves, and other organs.

Although currently there is no cure or prevention for RA, a lot can be done to help manage the condition. A variety of treatments exist to treat the symptoms, and they can result in less pain and stiffness with easier movement.

☆ Exercise helps lessen symptoms of RA and can make you feel better overall. Appropriate and moderate stretching and strengthening will help relieve the pain and keep the muscles and tendons around affected joints flexible and strong. Low impact exercises such as swimming, walking, water aerobics, and stationary bicycling can all reduce pain while helping to maintain strength, flexibility, and cardiovascular function. Physical therapists can teach you other techniques to manage the pain and restore joint motion and muscle strength.

☆ Weight control for people with RA usually means trying to maintain a recommended, healthy weight. People with RA are generally not overweight. Of greater concern are anemia and weight loss.

☆ It is crucial that people with rheumatoid arthritis take charge of their health. Pain and symptoms are definitely worsened by stress, exhaustion, over-activity, poor diet, and lack of sleep. A healthy routine appears to have positive effects on RA. If you are diagnosed with RA, it is imperative that you learn all you can about the disease so that you can take action to prevent its crippling effects.

Gout

Gout is a condition in which uric acid exceeds normal levels. Rather than being flushed by the kidneys through the urine, the uric acid forms crystals that deposit in the joints. These deposits result in inflammation, causing pain, swelling, redness, and tenderness.

Gout is predominantly a disease of adult men. In fact, it is the most common cause of inflammatory arthritis in men over age forty, and men have at least four times greater likelihood of developing gout than women. Women rarely develop gout before reaching menopause.

The onset of gout is usually quick and unexpected. Often, people who develop gout will do so during the night while sleeping. During the night, they are awakened by acute pain in the big toe or, more rarely, in the heel, ankle, or instep. There is also a pressure and tightness around the area, and sometimes the pain becomes quite severe. Gout typically affects the joint at the base of the big toe. In over half of all initial attacks, this is the first joint affected though almost any other joint can be affected.

The majority of initial gout attacks involve only one joint and, with treatment, subside within three to ten days. Over fifty percent of people who have had an acute attack of gout will have a recurrence within the year. Over time the attacks may become more frequent, longer lasting, and often involve more joints. A number of factors seem to contribute to gout. Acute gout may be triggered by events such as surgery, heart attacks, or trauma. Use of alcohol or some medications, such as certain diuretics, particularly those used to treat high blood pressure, can set off a gout attack. Such foods as seafood and liver and drinks such as coffee and tea may contribute to gout because they may cause your body to produce too much uric acid.

If you suffer from gout attacks, reduce your intake of coffee, cocoa, chocolate, and tea. You should also avoid certain animal proteins, including seafood, liver, kidney, heart, gizzard, sweetbreads, meat extracts, and gravy. Some vegetables may also present a problem. These include peas, beans, spinach, and lentils. Alcohol (beer, wine, etc.) also stops uric acid from leaving the body and can trigger gout. Sudden changes in diet or dramatic weight gain/loss may also cause gout attacks.

Heat or cold application can provide temporary relief of pain. Heat helps to reduce pain and stiffness by relaxing aching muscles and increasing circulation to the area. There is some concern, however, that heat may worsen the symptoms in an already inflamed joint. Cold helps numb the area by constricting the blood vessels and blocking nerve impulses in the joint. Applying ice or cold packs is very helpful in decreasing inflammation.

> *Drinking a quart of organic cherry juice will help eliminate the crystals in the joints.*

Lupus

Like rheumatoid arthritis, lupus is an autoimmune disease. It affects men, women, and children, but it occurs most often in women of childbearing age. Lupus is actually the name given to a group of chronic autoimmune diseases. Systemic lupus erythematosus (SLE) is the most common and serious type of lupus. With SLE, the immune system begins to malfunction, generating antibodies that attack healthy tissue. As a result, the tissue becomes inflamed. This can occur in the skin, muscles, joints, heart, lungs, kidneys, blood vessels, and the nervous system. SLE fluctuates between periods of illness and remission.

Other types of lupus are discoid lupus erythematosus (DLE) and subacute cutaneous lupus (SCLE). With these types of lupus, skin rashes and sun sensitivity are the main symptoms, and the internal organs are not attacked. Approximately ten percent of those diagnosed with these more limited forms of lupus will, however, go on to develop symptoms of SLE.

As in other forms of arthritis, diet can play a key role. Poor nutrition can bring on lupus attacks while a well-balanced diet can help to prevent them. Alcohol should be avoided altogether as it is known to contribute to flare-ups.

You Don't Have to Take It Lying Down

Lifestyle is a tremendous factor in reducing the pain and discomfort of all forms of arthritis. A healthy diet, supplementation, exercise, and some therapies can be extremely beneficial.

- Eat a diet low in fat that includes an abundance of fresh fruits and vegetables. Organic is always preferable, but in the case of arthritis, organic is definitely best. It is important to expose the immune system to as few toxins as possible.

- Avoid dairy, fried (greasy) foods, alcohol, caffeine, and sugar.

- Avoid allergy foods such as wheat, rye, corn, eggs, chocolate.

Exercise strengthens joints and connective tissue, increases circulation, and helps to activate the immune system. Light load-bearing exercise such as lifting free weights and low-impact exercises such as walking, swimming, and cycling are best for arthritis sufferers. Stretching is imperative prior to any activity. Therapies such as massage, therapeutic baths, and dry sauna may also offer relief from arthritis pain and stiffness.

Supplements are known to play an important and positive role in treating arthritis. In a recent study, glucosamine sulfate was shown to be effective in relieving the pain associated with osteoarthritis. Glucosamine has cartilage-rebuilding properties so, unlike anti-inflammatory drugs and analgesics, it treats the underlying cause of arthritis rather than just the symptoms.

> *The combination of glucosamine, chondroitin and Green-Lipped mussel is particularly effective, especially when taken continuously for several weeks.* **Ultimate Living** *offers our* **Arthritis Formula** *which contains all three: Green-Lipped mussel (especially effective in reducing inflammation) combined with glucosamine and chondroitin.*

Arthritis, particularly the autoimmune forms such as rheumatoid and lupus, is greatly exacerbated by stress and lack of rest. Proper rest is crucial to staving off arthritic attacks. Learning to rest and relax will act as a natural pain-killer. Deep breathing is great for relaxation, plus it fills the body with oxygen that is vital in increasing circulation and helping the body to expel certain toxins.

Once again, if you take care of your immune system, it will help take care of you.

Chapter Eleven

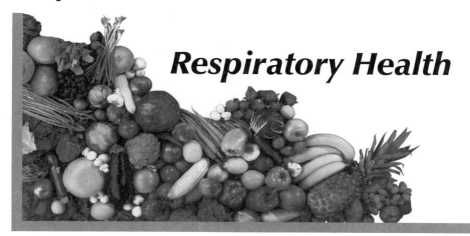

Respiratory Health

R espiratory disease is on the rise. More and more children and adults are diagnosed with asthma, chronic obstructive pulmonary disease (COPD), and chronic bronchitis each year. More than thirty-five million Americans are living with such chronic lung diseases as asthma, emphysema, and chronic bronchitis.

Think of the lungs as your body's cleaning crew. These pink, spongy organs cycle air by taking in oxygen and then removing carbon dioxide gas as waste when you exhale. Your lungs also protect against dust particles and other irritants that you inhale by using tiny hairs called cilia to sweep the material up to your throat where you can cough it out. In people with lung disease, the cilia and other parts of the lungs are damaged.

At rest, the average adult breathes in and out between twelve and eighteen times a minute. Surprisingly, only about ten percent of the air in the lungs is actually changed with each cycle of inhaling and exhaling, but up to eighty percent can be exchanged in rigorous exercise.

The lungs include the lobes, lobules, bronchi, bronchioles, infundibula, and alveoli or air sacs. The lungs actually contain 300 million alveoli, and their respiratory surface is equal to about 756 square feet for the exchange of gases. More than just inflatable airbags, the lungs perform a complex interaction for the body's cardiovascular and respiratory systems–bringing in air (oxygen) to be absorbed by the bloodstream while removing the carbon dioxide.

The cardiovascular and respiratory systems participate equally in respiration to provide the body with oxygen and to expel waste gases. The respiratory system provides for gas exchange, whereas the cardiovascular system transports gases in the blood between the lungs and the cells.

Air Quality

The problem is that the air we breathe has become increasingly detrimental to our lung health. As ozone levels and air pollution problems rise, so do the numbers of individuals with respiratory difficulties and disease.

Ozone is a form of oxygen. It results primarily from the reaction of sunlight with hydrocarbons and nitrogen oxides emitted in fuel combustion (automobiles). Ozone oxidizes when it comes in contact with body tissues such as those in the lung. It acts as a powerful respiratory irritant at levels frequently found in urban areas, especially during the summer months. Ozone exposure can lead to shortness of breath, chest pain when inhaling deeply, wheezing, and coughing.

> *Ground level ozone (man-made) in the lower atmosphere is not the same as the natural layer of ozone in the upper atmosphere which protects us from the sun's ultraviolet rays.*

Long term exposure to ozone may lead to reduced lung function, inflammation of the lung lining, and increased respiratory malfunction and discomfort. The EPA has listed three groups of people at particular risk from ozone exposure: people with pre-existing respiratory disease such as asthma, chronic bronchitis, and emphysema; individuals who exercise outdoors; and people who are highly sensitive to ozone.

"Americans need to know about unhealthy air pollution in their communities," says John L. Kirkwood, American Lung Association President and Chief Executive Officer. According to Kirkwood, "The threat may be invisible to the human eye, but it is real—and it can kill."

For the first time, the American Lung Association's annual State of the Air report uses data from a new national air-quality surveillance network to go beyond its traditional analysis of smog, or ozone air pollution, to include particle pollution. Produced by power plant emissions, diesel exhaust, and wood burning, among other sources, particle pollution can be dangerous both when it reaches unhealthy levels over a few hours or a few days and with constant daily exposure over a long period of time.

Both particle pollution and ozone threaten air quality. While particle pollution emerges as a widespread problem affecting a quarter of all Americans, ozone levels continue to endanger nearly half the nation (136 million Americans).

Here are some of the cities and counties most affected by the poorest air quality:

> **Northeast** - New York City, Philadelphia, Harrisburg, Pittsburgh, Washington, DC, Newark, Bridgeport, and Baltimore

> **Southeast** - Atlanta, Birmingham, Knoxville, Louisville, Charleston, Raleigh-Durham, and Winston-Salem

> **Midwest** - Chicago, Cleveland, Cincinnati, St. Louis, and Detroit

> **Southwest** - Dallas-Ft. Worth, Houston, and Phoenix

> **West** - Los Angeles, San Diego, San Francisco, Sacramento, Fresno, Eugene, Seattle, Provo, and Salt Lake City

The complex and dangerous health effects of particle pollution were confirmed in a National Research Council report released in March 2004.

- Twenty-eight percent (more than 81 million) of the U.S. population lives in areas with unhealthy short-term levels of particle pollution.

- Nearly one-quarter of Americans (66 million) live in areas with unhealthy year-round levels of particle pollution.

- Nearly half of all Americans (136 million) live in counties with unhealthy levels of ozone despite substantial reductions in ozone in the thirty-four years spent fighting the problem.

- All totaled, some 159 million Americans live in counties with unhealthy levels of either ozone or periodic to year-round levels of particle pollution.

- Most alarmingly, 46 million Americans live in counties where all three levels are unhealthy.

Asthma

Asthma is a reversible obstructive lung disease, caused by an increased reaction of the airways to various stimuli. It is a chronic inflammatory condition with acute exacerbations. Asthma can be life-threatening if not properly managed.

Asthma breathing problems usually happen in episodes, but the inflammation underlying the condition is continuous. An asthma episode is a series of events that result in narrowed airways. These include swelling of the lining, tightening of the muscle, and increased secretion of mucus in the airway. The narrowing of the airways is responsible for the difficulty in breathing and the telltale wheeze.

Despite the number of medications available today, asthma is still poorly controlled. A recent survey found that forty-eight percent of people with asthma say that the disease limits their ability to take part in sports and recreation, thirty-six percent say that it limits their normal physical exertion, and twenty-five percent say that it actually interferes with their social activities.

Asthma is characterized by excessive sensitivity of the lungs to stimuli. Triggers can range from viral infections to allergies, irritating gases, and particles in the air.

Everyone reacts differently to the various triggers that include the following:

- Respiratory infections, colds

- Cigarette smoke

- Allergic reactions to such allergens as pollen, mold, animal dander, feathers, dust, certain foods, and cockroaches

- Indoor and outdoor pollutants, including ozone

- Exposure to cold air or sudden temperature changes

- Excitement/stress

- Exercise

Chronic Bronchitis

The bronchi are air passages connecting the windpipe (trachea) with the sacs of the lung (alveoli) where oxygen is taken up by the blood. Bronchitis is an inflammation of the bronchi causing excessive mucus production and swelling of the bronchial walls.

Many people suffer a brief attack of acute bronchitis with fever, coughing, and spitting when they have a severe cold. Chronic bronchitis, however, is the term applied when the coughing and spitting continue for months and recur each year, generally lasting slightly longer each time. Undue breathlessness with exertion eventually occurs due to obstruction to air flow in the air passages caused by swelling of the bronchial wall and the presence of mucus that cannot be cleared.

Cigarette smoking is the most common cause of chronic bronchitis, which rarely occurs in the non-smoker. Inhaled tobacco products impair the ability of the lungs to combat infections. Environmental pollution may also contribute to the development of chronic bronchitis.

The patient with advanced bronchitis may be unable to walk or climb stairs without supplemental oxygen and may even be limited to sitting in a chair or lying in bed because of shortness of breath. There is also a type of heart failure that may develop in the late stages of this disease. Even minor chest infections can send a person suffering from advanced chronic bronchitis to the hospital.

The best treatment for chronic bronchitis is prevention, which means no smoking. People suffering with chronic bronchitis should avoid excessive dust and fumes.

Regular exercise is very important for patients suffering from chronic bronchitis. Exercise does not improve the ability of the lungs to take up oxygen, but the effects of physical fitness on the cardiovascular system will compensate somewhat for the impaired lung function.

Emphysema

Emphysema is a condition in which the walls between the alveoli or air sacs within the lungs lose their ability to stretch and recoil. The air sacs become weakened and break. Elasticity of the lung tissue is lost, causing air to be trapped in the air sacs and impairing the exchange of oxygen and carbon dioxide. Also, the support of the airways is lost, allowing for airflow obstruction.

Emphysema begins with the destruction of air sacs (alveoli) in the lungs where oxygen from the air is exchanged for carbon dioxide in the blood. The walls of the air sacs become thin and fragile. Damage to the air sacs is irreversible and results in permanent "holes" in the tissues of the lower lungs. As air sacs are destroyed, the lungs are able to transfer less and less oxygen to the bloodstream, causing shortness of breath. The lungs also lose their elasticity, which is important in keeping airways open. The patient experiences great difficulty exhaling.

Symptoms of emphysema include shortness of breath, cough, and limited exercise tolerance. Over 3.1 million Americans have been diagnosed with emphysema, of which ninety-one percent were 45 years of age or older. Men tend to have higher rates of emphysema than women.

Emphysema comes on very gradually. Years of exposure to the irritation of cigarette smoke usually precede its development. A person may initially visit the doctor because he or she has begun to feel shortness of breath during activity or exercise. As the disease progresses, a brief walk can be enough to bring on difficulty in breathing. Some people may have had chronic bronchitis before developing emphysema.

Some patients benefit from oxygen therapy, either when exercising or on a nearly continuous basis. Physicians may emphasize the importance of regular exercise to maintain physical fitness and even refer a patient with emphysema to a respiratory rehabilitation program.

Chronic Obstructive Pulmonary Disease (COPD)

Chronic obstructive pulmonary disease (COPD) is a group of chronic lung diseases that make breathing difficult. COPD is often a mix of two diseases, chronic bronchitis and emphysema.

In COPD, airflow through the airways leading to and within the lungs (bronchial tubes) is partially blocked, resulting in difficulty in breathing. As the disease gets worse, breathing becomes more labored, and it may become arduous to carry out everyday activities. There is currently no cure for COPD, but there are things you can do to improve your quality of life.

When you have COPD, you may be more susceptible to lung infections. Washing your hands often and thoroughly is an easy way to ward off infection. Also, try to avoid close contact with people who have colds or the flu.

Exercising regularly can build your strength and improve your outlook. There are also breathing exercises that may help to improve your lung function.

Chronic Sinusitis

Chronic sinusitis usually coincides with a history of allergies or exposure to respiratory irritants. It is marked by degenerative changes in the sinus membranes that impair proper sinus drainage. The best way to alleviate sinusitis is to minimize exposure to the offending allergens or irritants.

Persons suffering with chronic sinusitis need to filter the air at their home with good quality air filters. High Efficiency Particulate Air (HEPA) filters are effective in removing pollen, dust, animal dander, and other particulates.

The household dust mite is one of the worst offenders for people with sinusitis and respiratory conditions. They proliferate in carpets, upholstery, and bed linens. Limiting fabric surfaces and carpeting and regularly washing linens in hot water will help minimize dust mites.

In addition, it is important to be tested for food allergies and to make every effort to remove the allergens from the diet. The worst offenders are milk, eggs, corn, wheat, chocolate, and some citrus fruits, particularly oranges.

Antioxidants that support immune function are necessary to help prevent infections caused by the chronic irritation of sinusitis and respiratory disease. Oral enzyme supplements have been used to treat chronic sinusitis for over thirty years. Bromelain, an enzyme from pineapple that breaks up proteins, has been shown to relieve swelling and redness of the nasal membranes and seems to have a thinning action on the overproduction of mucus.

Ultimate Living Aloe-Papaya Drink *is a rich source of bromelain.*

Lifestyle for Lung Health

Nutrition

Green leafy vegetables are especially good for people suffering with lung disease, mainly because they contain high levels of magnesium, which is excellent for relaxing constricted bronchial muscles.

It is especially important to drink plenty of water to reduce mucus secretions. Water with lemon is especially beneficial. It is best to avoid dairy products as they cause excess mucus production. Limit starchy foods and sodium and avoid soft drinks, greasy and fried foods, MSG, sulfites, caffeine, and sugary foods.

If you are asthmatic, it is a good idea to be tested for food allergies so you will know what foods might trigger attacks.

Persons with lung disease should eat six smaller meals instead of three big meals. Many people with chronic lung disease feel more shortness of breath when their stomach is full. This is because the diaphragm cannot work as well when the stomach is full. You can satisfy your nutritional needs, keep your stomach comfortable, and help your diaphragm to work better by eating smaller, more frequent meals.

Chronic lung disease, including asthma, is often treated with steroids, either orally or inhaled. Steroids are strong medicines that decrease swollen airways. They also have some nutritional side effects such as interfering with the way the body uses some nutrients.

If you are being treated with steroids, it is very important to eat a well balanced diet that includes foods from each food group and to drink plenty of pure water. Over a long period of time, steroids can increase the risk of osteoporosis. It is, therefore, very important to eat foods high in calcium. Since dairy tends to increase mucus production, you need to obtain calcium from other food sources.

Many foods other than milk and milk products contain calcium, for example, certain green vegetables (such as broccoli and kale) and some canned fish with small bones (such as sardines). Other foods have calcium added to them, including juices, soy milk, tofu, and some foods made with lime (calcium carbonate).

Ultimate Living Cal-Mag Plus *is an excellent source of calcium.*

Antioxidants are valuable nutrients for lung health. They fight the free radicals that cause lung tissue inflammation and oxidation. Antioxidants such as vitamin E are found in foods such as olive and vegetable oil, seeds and nuts. Vitamin C is found in fruits and vegetables, and beta-carotene in yellow, orange, and dark green vegetables such as pumpkin, carrots, and spinach.

Exercise

People with lung disease often feel like they are struggling just to breathe, so the idea of exercise seems impossible. Regular exercise, however, can have very positive benefits both physically and psychologically for the person suffering with such a disease. Exercise also helps by strengthening leg and arm muscles and building endurance, which reduces breathlessness over time and greatly improves stamina.

Regular activity also serves to reduce the depression and anxiety that often accompany lung disease.

Walking is one of the best exercises for people with lung disease. Yoga, tai chi, and other activities that emphasize breathing techniques and balanced movements are also very beneficial. Swimming is great for people with asthma. The moisture on the surface of the water seems to help ward off an asthma attack sometimes brought on by exertion.

Everyone should avoid exercising outdoors when air quality is bad, particularly people with lung disease. Air pollution can even hurt people who do not have lung disease. Exercise makes everyone more vulnerable to health damage from air pollutants because, when we exercise, we draw more air into the lungs, exposing them to more harmful pollutants. We also breathe mostly through the mouth, bypassing the nose (the body's first line of defense against pollutants).

Pay attention to pollution levels especially in the summer when ozone levels are at their highest. Ozone air pollution, a main component of smog, is worse from May to October. Since sunlight contributes to the formation of smog, exercising in the morning can also help reduce exposure. When air pollution levels are high outdoors, it is best to exercise inside.

Air quality is always worse near freeways, busy streets, and industrial areas.

Supplements

Researchers now say that taking antioxidant supplements can help reduce the effects of ozone pollution on lung health. Supplements may also help the body prevent and even reverse damage from toxins and pollutants.

Vitamin A and vitamin C are both powerful antioxidants and immune-system boosters, and both lead the charge in the battle against damaging free radicals.

Magnesium is excellent in helping relax constricted lung muscles and may make breathing easier. Dietary deficiencies in potassium and magnesium have been associated with impaired lung function.

Zinc and selenium may have some effect in reducing the severity of upper respiratory tract infections.

Studies have also shown that antioxidants may enhance lung function. The carotenoids lutein and zeaxanthin may be more effective in enhancing lung health than other antioxidants.

Omega-3 fatty acids, found in cold water oily fish and in supplements, have anti-inflammatory effects that may relieve bronchial inflammation.

*Ultimate Living Lung Formula specifically addresses the symptoms of lung disease. Our **Lung Formula** was developed to prevent and relieve all lung and respiratory problems. We have received many testimonies from people all over the country in appreciation of the improvement in their lung health. Try it! We believe you will experience the same results.*

What More You Can Do

As much as possible, a patient should avoid exposure to airborne irritants, including hair sprays, aerosol products, paint sprayers, and insecticides.

To minimize the amount of contaminants in the home, the following may be helpful measures:

- Ventilate by keeping windows open (weather permitting), by using exhaust fans for stoves and vents for furnaces, and by keeping fireplace flues open.

- Make sure wood-burning stoves or fireplaces are well ventilated and meet the Environmental Protection Agency's safety standards, and burn pressed wood products labeled "exterior grade" since they contain the least amount of pollutants from resins.

- Have furnaces and chimneys inspected and cleaned periodically.

- Eliminate molds and mildews stemming from household water damage.

- People who are sensitive to allergens, such as pollen, pet dander, house dust, and mold, should avoid exposure to them.

- Invest in a high quality HEPA (High Efficiency Particulate Air) filtering system for your home if possible, but at least for your sleeping area.

Quitting smoking is the first and most essential step in treating chronic obstructive lung disease and slowing its progress. In many people who quit, lung function stabilizes and eventually declines at about the rate of nonsmokers in the same age group. In some people, lung function may even improve slightly after quitting.

Respiratory infections can be very dangerous to persons already suffering from chronic lung diseases. It is crucial to keep your immune system in good working order. (Refer to Chapter One)

As with other chronic disorders, it is important to get proper rest and to avoid stress. Most of us experience stress at some point in our lives; but for people with asthma, stress and anxiety can be significant triggers for attacks. Try to avoid situations that cause stress. Practice effective time-management skills, setting priorities, and taking time out for yourself.

Chapter Twelve

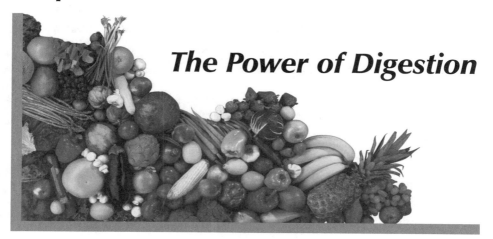

The Power of Digestion

D igestion is the process by which food and drink are broken down into their smallest parts so that the body can use them to build and nourish cells and to provide energy. Most of our immune system is focused on the digestive system. If we want to be healthy, it is imperative that we have a healthy digestive tract.

Commonly Used Terms:

▷ **Dyspepsia** is another name for indigestion.

▷ **Gastroesophageal reflux disease (GERD)** is a disorder of the lower end of the esophagus caused by stomach acid flowing backward into the esophagus and irritating the tissues.

▷ **Heartburn** is a popular term for an uncomfortable feeling in the stomach and lower esophagus, sometimes caused by the reflux of small amounts of stomach acid.

▷ **Peptic ulcer disease** is a stomach disorder marked by corrosion of the stomach lining due to acid in the stomach juices.

▷ **Reflux** is the backward flow of a body fluid or secretion. Indigestion is sometimes caused by the reflux of stomach acid into the esophagus.

> ➢ **Irritable bowel syndrome (IBS)** is an intestinal disorder that causes abdominal pain or discomfort, cramping or bloating, and diarrhea or constipation. Irritable bowel syndrome is a long-term but manageable condition.

> ➢ **Digestive enzymes** are complex protein molecules especially tailored to break down foods into nutrients that your body can then readily digest.

There are many symptoms of an inefficient digestive tract, including gas and stomach bloating, poor digestion, bad breath, lower backache, fatigue, body odor, and sallow skin. There are also many factors that can adversely affect the digestive tract.

These include:

- Eating too few live foods (fresh fruits and vegetables)
- Not drinking enough water
- Lack of sufficient enzyme activity
- Constipation
- Stress
- Certain medications
- Overuse of antibiotics

Classifications of Digestive Disorders

Doctors classify digestive disorders into several groups.

> ☆ Esophagitis is an inflammation of the esophagus. The esophagus carries food from the throat to the stomach. When it becomes irritated, especially by the reverse flow of stomach acid (reflux), a

person will experience intense heartburn. If this condition becomes chronic, the person may be diagnosed with gastroesophageal reflux disease (GERD). While antacids may give relief to heartburn, if the condition becomes chronic, you must seek medical attention as GERD can be the precursor to more serious esophageal disease.

☆ GERD is becoming more and more common, presently affecting over thirty percent of adult Americans. People who experience occasional heartburn that is relieved by taking antacids have indigestion of the peptic ulcer type, which is marked by corrosion of the stomach lining due to acid in the stomach juices. People with peptic ulcer type indigestion are often found to have a bacteria called Helicobacter pylori (H. Pylori) living in their stomach tissues and causing irritation of the lining of the stomach walls. Smokers or people over the age of 45 are the most likely group to have peptic ulcer disease.

☆ Most cases of chronic indigestion are of a nonulcer type. Nonulcer type indigestion is caused by abnormalities in the way the stomach empties its contents into the intestine or irregular stomach contractions. Young people appear to be the most vulnerable, probably due to lifestyle choices such as poor diet, alcohol consumption, lack of rest, and stress.

Indigestion

Take a look on the shelves of your local drugstore. It is obvious by the array of antacids and stomach-soothing medications that almost everyone at some time suffers from indigestion or a sour-stomach. Indigestion or dyspepsia is a widespread condition, estimated to occur in twenty-five percent of American adults. Most people with indigestion do not feel sick enough to see a doctor; nonetheless, it is a common reason for office visits. About three percent of visits to primary care physicians are for indigestion. Gas, bloating, indigestion, and heartburn are all symptoms of digestive distress. Many factors may contribute to these discomforts, most typically the type of food eaten or a lack of enzymes to properly break down and assimilate these foods.

Symptoms associated with indigestion have a variety of possible physical causes, ranging from food items to serious disorders. Milk, milk products, alcohol, tea, and coffee can cause indigestion because in some individuals they stimulate the production of acid. Some medications and prescription drugs can cause an irritation of the stomach lining. These include medicines such as aspirin, some antibiotics, steroids, iron supplements, oral contraceptives, and some antidepressants.

Chronic indigestion can also signal a number of illnesses such as disorders of the pancreas and gallbladder. In rare cases, indigestion suggests the presence of parasites. Pregnant women often complain of indigestion. Systemic disorders such as diabetes, thyroid disease, vascular disease, and cancer of the digestive tract may have indigestion as a symptom. Most serious is cancer of the digestive tract.

Indigestion frequently accompanies an emotional upset because the nervous system has an impact on the digestive tract. Some people have digestive systems that respond more dramatically to situations that make them nervous or upset and have more intense symptoms, including stomach cramps or even diarrhea.

Simple Things You Can Do to Prevent Indigestion:

- Stop smoking
- Cut down or eliminate alcohol consumption
- Limit your intake of coffee and tea
- Avoid fatty foods
- Avoid spicy foods

- Do not drink sodas

- Practice deep breathing

- Do not take medicine or aspirin on an empty stomach

- Lose weight

- Take digestive enzymes

> ***Ultimate Living Complete Enzymes*** contain food enzymes, digestive enzymes, and metabolic enzymes. These three classes of enzymes are all important to break down fats, starches, sugars, protein, and fiber.

Irritable Bowel Syndrome

Irritable bowel syndrome (IBS) is an intestinal disorder that causes abdominal pain or discomfort, cramping or bloating, and diarrhea or constipation. Irritable bowel syndrome is a long-term but manageable condition, and it is one of the most common intestinal disorders. Although most people's symptoms are so mild that they never see a doctor for treatment, some people may have troublesome symptoms, especially abdominal cramps, bloating, and diarrhea.

Malabsorption

Another common digestive tract problem that may not be associated with any specific symptoms is malabsorption. Up to thirty percent of adults simply cannot absorb essential nutrients, particularly the B vitamins and minerals. Diarrhea, bloating or cramping, frequent bulky stools, muscle wasting, and a distended abdomen may accompany malabsorption. Prolonged malabsorption can result in malnutrition and vitamin deficiencies.

Constipation

One of the most frequent bowel problems people experience is constipation. Constipation is generally attributed to a low fiber diet and lack of sufficient water, both of which cause our fecal matter to become condensed and compressed.

A constipated system is one in which the time that toxic wastes remain in the bowel is too long. Often the consistency of the stool can cause strain, which over time may cause hemorrhoids, varicose veins, hiatal hernia, or other problems induced by straining. The longer the toxic waste matter sits in our bowel, the more proteins are allowed to putrefy, fats to become rancid, and carbohydrates to ferment.

The longer your body is exposed to putrefying food in your intestines, the greater the risk of developing disease. Even with one bowel movement per day, you will still have at least two meals worth of waste matter putrefying in your colon at all times. On top of all this, your system can also become continuously self-polluting due to the poisonous gases caused by foods you do not tolerate. These poisonous gases can enter your bloodstream, irritating your organs and joints. Alternating between constipation and diarrhea or having diarrhea alone are also indications of foul matter in your intestines. Finally, the much more serious problems of cancer and immune system dysfunctions begin with a toxic bowel.

The long held belief of some health professionals is that many people just have fewer bowel movements than others. Although this may be true, the professionals have neglected to inform such individuals that, consequently, they are very likely harboring a fertile breeding ground for serious diseases and possibly death. Infrequent or poor quality bowel movements over an extended period of time are very hazardous to your health.

> *Ideally, you should have a bowel movement after each meal.*

Ways to Prevent Constipation:

- Drink eight or more glasses of water a day—add lemon for even better cleansing effects.

- Eat a diet high in fiber-rich foods.

- Limit your intake of dairy products.

- Eliminate high-fat, fried, greasy, or sugary foods from your diet.

> **Ultimate Living Fiber Cleanse** will help you have regular bowel movements and will eliminate bowel toxins.

Diverticulitis

Diverticulitis is a condition in which the lining of the colon becomes inflamed and results in the forming of small pouch-like areas called diverticula where waste matter can become trapped. When this happens, the painful condition diverticulitis occurs with symptoms such as fever, chills, and pain. Poor diet, stress, and smoking can bring on an attack.

Americans and people living in other developed countries are at the greatest risk of contracting diverticulitis because they consume diets deficient in fiber. A diet low in fiber puts a strain on the colon and its ability to remove waste. Ultimately, the strain will cause the pouches or diverticula to form. This condition can be quite painful and sometimes dangerous, particularly when the diverticula rupture, spilling waste and bacteria into the bloodstream.

Consume an adequate amount of fiber and drink plenty of water. Eat a low-carbohydrate diet, high in protein from fish and vegetable sources rather than from red meat. Eat plenty of green, leafy vegetables and lots of garlic (for its healing and detoxifying properties). Never let yourself become constipated.

Fiber, Fiber, and More Fiber

Fiber is the portion of foods that does not break down when passing through the digestive tract. Since these substances have such a large impact on overall health, individuals are encouraged to eat fiber-rich foods. Fiber is known to lower the risk for such diseases as colorectal cancers, gallstones, diabetes, breast cancer, and heart disease, among others.

There are two types of fiber: soluble and insoluble. Soluble fiber dissolves during digestion and creates a gel-like substance that protects the entire digestive tract from absorbing various substances and, at the same time, prevents or reduces the absorption of certain substances into the bloodstream from the intestines. Also, when mixed with liquid, this gel helps produce a softer stool. One of the substances soluble fiber helps to protect against is cholesterol. By reducing the rate at which cholesterol is absorbed, soluble fiber serves as an important weapon against heart disease. By regulating the rate of glucose absorption, thus reducing drastic variations in blood sugar levels, it also aids in controlling diabetes. Soluble fiber is found in fruits, vegetables, seeds, brown rice, barley, oats, and oat bran.

Insoluble fiber enters and exits the digestive tract without being significantly altered. It also absorbs water and, as a result, prevents constipation and aids regular waste elimination. When waste is expelled from the body regularly, the time that potentially harmful substances remain in the colon is lessened. Research has also shown that insoluble fiber lowers the risk for breast cancer by combining with estrogen through digestion and thus reducing the level of estrogen in the body. Insoluble fiber is like a sponge; it absorbs water and moves solid waste out of the intestines. It is found mainly in whole grains and on the outside of seeds, fruits, and legumes. Other sources of insoluble fiber are wheat, beans, bran, figs, and artichokes.

A major advantage of a high-fiber diet is its effect on weight control. Studies have shown that the majority of seriously overweight people have diets low in foods containing fiber. Since fiber-rich foods are filling and, for the most part, low in fat, individuals are satisfied with less food and lose weight easily.

Although dietary fiber is a type of carbohydrate that is not digested, it remains an essential part of a healthy diet. It is recommended that between twenty-five and thirty-five grams of fiber be consumed daily, yet the majority of us get only half the recommended amount. For children over the age of two, a simple rule of thumb is the child's age plus five equals the grams of fiber needed daily. This is not difficult if fruits, vegetables, and grains are part of the daily diet. In addition, at least eight glasses of water should be consumed daily to aid the movement of food through the digestive tract. A diet rich in fiber may help to manage and protect against numerous diseases and also promote regular bowel movements.

Both soluble and insoluble fibers are important in helping to maintain regular bowel movements. Insoluble fiber prevents and manages problems such as constipation and hemorrhoids by producing a larger, softer stool that passes through the digestive system more quickly and easily. In addition, complications from intestinal diseases such as diverticulosis or irritable bowel syndrome (IBS) are prevented by a diet rich in high fiber foods.

Focus on choosing a variety of the high fiber foods listed below and you will not be caught reading in the bathroom because of constipation.

Blackberries	Spinach	Brazil nuts
Raspberries	Beet greens	Peanuts
Strawberries	Kale	Walnuts
Rye	Collard	Cherries
Broccoli	Swiss chard	Brussel sprouts
Green beans	Turnip greens	Stone ground whole wheat
Apples with skin	Almonds	

Your digestive system is only a part of your body's amazing detoxifying system. Exercise is beneficial not only to get the digestive system moving but also to promote perspiration, another way the body rids itself of toxins and wastes. Also, when you exercise, you breathe harder and more deeply, allowing your lungs to expel undesirable wastes as well. Plus your circulatory system gets moving, thus assisting the bloodstream to cleanse itself.

A combinination of good diet, exercise, plenty of water, and supplements such as digestive enzymes should give your body the opportunity to cleanse itself regularly. With a healthier digestive system, you will almost immediately notice an improvement in your complexion, your energy levels, even your sleeping habits. You may even notice fewer colds and viruses since you will also be giving your immune system a rest.

> *Also, don't forget to add* **Ultimate Living Green Miracle** *and* **Aloe-Papaya Drink** *t*o *your diet. They contain all the required servings of fruits and vegetables, and they promote good elimination.*

Digestive Enzymes

Digestive enzymes are protein molecules specially tailored to break down foods into nutrients that your body can then readily digest. The human body produces some twenty-two different digestive enzymes, and many more are found in fruits, vegetables, meats, grains, and other foods. When you eat a meal, digestive enzymes that are released from your salivary glands, stomach, and small intestine immediately get to work to speed up the digestive process. Each enzyme acts on a specific type of food. A variety of different proteases, for example, break down the components of protein. Amylases help digest carbohydrates; lipases break down fats; and cellulases, found in plants, digest fiber.

Chapter Twelve: The Power of Digestion

Many people are lacking enzymes because of inadequate diets, over-refined foods, environmental toxins, and poor health. We are all born with enough enzymes to last for the rest of our lives. However, our Standard American Diet (SAD), complete with its abundance of preservatives, mineral deficient foods, as well as environmental factors, deplete our bodies of their enzyme reserves by age forty. Therefore, it is essential that we supplement our diets with digestive enzymes. Nearly all types of digestive problems can benefit from enzyme therapy. In the case of heartburn, for example, the thinking is that any means of accelerating the stomach's emptying of food may well reduce stomach acid and lessen irritation along the digestive tract. Conditions such as irritable bowel syndrome or inflammatory bowel disease (Crohn's disease, ulcerative colitis) may also be relieved. Digestive enzymes aid in the absorption of valuable nutrients, thus preventing malabsorption.

Digestive enzyme supplements are often used in natural treatment for the symptoms of various ailments, from simple heartburn and bloating to more persistent problems such as chronic indigestion and irritable bowel syndrome. Taking enzymes can aid in several functions. A good enzyme supplement can assist in optimizing elimination by breaking down carbohydrates, fats, proteins, and fiber. You will also be insuring better absorption of good nutrients.

Digestive problems often develop as we grow older because stores of digestive enzymes decline with advancing age. Taking supplemental enzymes helps to restore good digestion by replenishing these diminishing supplies. They are excellent in eliminating flatulence, heartburn, irritable bowel syndrome, and other digestive complaints.

If you're on anticoagulants or other blood-thinning medications, let your doctor know. Some enzymes, such as bromelain, can thin the blood further and possibly cause complications.

Wait a couple hours after taking digestive enzymes before taking an antacid since acid neutralizers (such as TUMS or Mylanta) may interfere with the activity of certain enzyme supplements. Eventually you should no longer need these types of drugs at all.

> # Remember!
>
> *Ultimate Living Complete Enzymes* *contain food enzymes, digestive enzymes, and metabolic enzymes. These three classes of enzymes are all important to break down fats, starches, sugars, protein, and fiber.*

Aloe Vera

Aloe vera eases heartburn, ulcers, and other types of digestive upset. A juice made from the aloe gel acts as an anti-inflammatory and can be taken internally as a remedy for certain digestive complaints. European folk medicine calls for using aloe vera juice to relieve heartburn and ulcers.

Trials indicate that aloe vera heals peptic ulcers, keeps intestinal secretions at normal levels, positively influences bowel flora, controls gastric and intestinal pH, and limits adverse bacteria in the colon, thus reducing putrefaction.

> *For heartburn: Drink one ounce of* **Ultimate Living Aloe-Papaya Drink** *two to four times a day.*

Acidophilus

Acidophilus is a vital and normal inhabitant of healthy human intestines. It can help to inhibit the growth of undesirable microorganisms entering the digestive system. In addition, research indicates acidophilus can improve the digestion of lactose and increase the body's ability to absorb and make use of vitamin B. Acidophilus is also effective in keeping the delicate balance of good versus bad bacteria in line, particularly when antibiotics have caused a disruption in the normal balance.

Cleanse Your Colon

In addition to constipation, another cause for gas and bloating is putrefied food and toxins left in the bowel. Many naturopaths and practitioners of natural medicine believe that all disease originates in the colon. Wastes left in the colon can be reabsorbed into the body and can tax the immune system so that bacteria, viruses, and other diseases have a fertile breeding ground.

There are several guidelines for proper elimination. Your stools should be nearly odorless, meaning that the time between stools is not so long that it gives waste products time to putrefy. Your stools should float, indicating an adequate supply of fiber. Your bowel movements should not require straining or pain. You should have a bowel movement everyday and ideally after every meal. While some people do not have a bowel movement everyday, you are technically constipated if you do not. If you suffer from gas and bloating, you may not be eliminating properly.

Numerous situations can cause constipation: a low-fiber diet or one with too much sugar, processed and fast foods, food allergies, and lack of exercise. Certain prescription drugs, particularly pain medications, are known to slow down the elimination process.

The person on a typical American diet retains seven or eight meals of undigested food and waste material in the colon. Nutrition experts recommend a good cleansing of the colon at least once annually.

*We recommend cleansing your colon each season (four times a year) by taking three **Ultimate Living Fiber Cleanse** capsules with an eight ounce glass of water each evening before bedtime for fifteen days.*

A good cleansing program should always begin by removing the waste in your colon, the last portion of your food processing chain. You should never attempt to detoxify your liver, blood, or lymph system without first cleansing the bowel. Otherwise, toxins will only get recycled back into your body. Different methods of colon cleansing include colon hydrotherapy (colonics), enemas, and herbal supplements.

The digestive system is your body's cleanser. If you keep it as clean as possible, your body and immune system will have less work to do. Proper diet and adequate activity are key. The slogan for your immune system health should be "Keep It Clean."

Chapter Thirteen

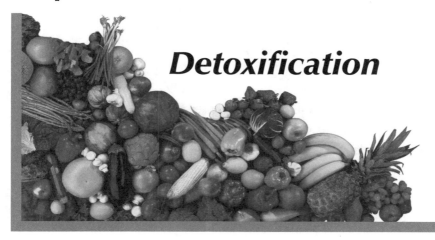

Detoxification

T hink of your garbage can. After trash has been sitting in it for a while, you can smell the results. When your body is full of toxins, it is like a garbage can that has not been emptied.

Toxins exist everywhere and can lead to serious health problems. They are in food and the environment, and they persist because of our insufficient metabolic ability to rid the body of all that we are exposed to on a daily basis. They can drain the body of energy and make you more susceptible to disease and infection. Toxins tend to concentrate in the liver and gastrointestinal tract, both of which are responsible for eliminating toxins from the body. Since everyone is exposed to toxins, all of us can use a detoxification treatment on a regular basis.

Think about a piece of sterling silver. If allowed to tarnish, it loses its luster, looks old, and may even deteriorate. If it is kept clean and polished, it looks bright and beautiful, plus it lasts a long time. The environment, particularly for those of us living urban lifestyles, is not working to keep us bright and beautiful. In fact, our environment is really tarnishing our body day in and day out.

We are constantly bombarded by toxins in the form of pesticides, hormones, and herbicides with which food and the soil are treated. Bacteria;

viruses; too much alcohol; coffee and other caffeine-containing drinks; smoking; and medications that have powerful effects on the liver, stomach, and other parts of the body can prove toxic.

We have got to make every effort to rid ourselves of as many toxins as possible, especially if, as many people believe, an overload causes us to feel tired, run-down, and even ill. Then we must (and this is imperative in the battle against disease and aging) keep our immune systems in top running order.

Maximizing our immune system is impossible if we are on "toxic overload."

Here are very easy steps to follow in detoxifying. In order to achieve optimum wellness and to feel as energetic as possible, these should become part of your lifestyle. Try these suggestions for two weeks, and you will see a marked difference in your elimination, energy levels, and overall appearance. The bonus is that you will also shed a few pounds.

> **Upon arising,** drink an eight-ounce glass of water with a splash of organic cranberry juice and a squeeze of lemon. Throughout the day, drink plenty of water. A good rule of thumb is to divide your weight in half and drink that many ounces of water a day. We mean good, clean, pure water, not tap water that is truly hardly fit to drink. For instance, if your weight is 140 pounds, you should drink at least 70 ounces of water per day. This is an easy addition to your lifestyle. Good bottled water is available everywhere, and there are great water filters you can add to your kitchen sink or refrigerator. To avoid "water fatigue," throw a piece of fruit (lemon, lime, orange segment, even berries) into your glass.

> **For breakfast,** have a piece of whole grain toast with all-fruit preserves (no added sugar) and half a cup of yogurt.

➤ **For a mid-morning snack,** have a cup of vegetable broth.

➤ **For lunch,** try to eat organic fresh fruits and vegetables. Salads, beans, fresh juices, stir-fried veggies cooked in a little good-quality olive oil, nuts, seeds, and yogurt are all wonderful for you and easy to obtain and prepare. The more organic food we eat, the healthier our bodies will be since we will be consuming fewer harmful chemicals. We recommend eating as many raw fruits and veggies as possible (no starches such as potatoes or corn). Steaming is a quick, easy, and healthy way of cooking vegetables. If you don't own a veggie steamer, get one (there are very inexpensive steamer baskets available). Recommendations are now nine to thirteen servings of fruits and vegetables per day. A serving is one-half cup.

> *Three scoops of **Ultimate Living Green Miracle** give you your daily supply of organic fruits and vegetables.*

➤ **For an afternoon snack,** have a piece of fruit and a cup of green tea.

> ***Green Miracle** is a great afternoon pick-me-up. If you choose to take **Green Miracle** in the afternoon, take 1½ scoops in the morning and 1½ scoops in the afternoon when you need a boost.*

➤ **For dinner,** select a lean protein coupled with steamed vegetables. Beans, lentils, eggs, chicken, fish (excluding shell fish), and a little lean red meat are good, but avoid fatty and fried foods.

> **Before bedtime,** have a cup of herbal tea (it contains no caffeine).

> **Avoid salt.** Instead of salt use fresh herbs, spices, chilies, and lemon juice to enhance the flavor of food. Salt causes fluid retention and does not allow the body to properly eliminate the very toxins we are working to expel.

> **Try to get as much rest as possible.** As your body starts to detoxify, you might feel a little out of sorts for a few days before you start reaping the benefits of your detoxification, which usually happens during the second week. You may even experience some skin break-outs or even a little stomach upset. This should all dissipate by the second week. Remember that the toxins have to come out somewhere. It may be through the skin, and certainly it will be through the bowel. The severity will depend on how toxic you have allowed your body to become, but these side effects are usually quite minimal. Once these effects are over, your skin will glow, and your stomach will not only be lots flatter but also lots healthier!

> **Try light exercise.** This increases lymph activity within the body, causing you to sweat and generate more urine, encouraging liver activity and stimulating elimination of waste products. Walking, swimming, and cycling are beneficial, but strenuous exercise is not advised when you are detoxifying your body.

> **Avoid stressful situations.** Stress releases toxic chemicals into our bodies. Stressful situations are never a good thing, but particularly avoid them while you are trying to cleanse your system.

> **Do we need to tell you not to smoke or drink alcohol?**

A Dietary Tip

Fruit should always be eaten on an empty stomach or fifteen minutes prior to eating a meal. Fruit is digested more quickly than other foods. If it is eaten after another food, it will putrefy in the stomach and keep food from digesting properly.

In the second week of detoxification, you may add whole grains and brown rice. When it comes to starchy foods, rather than eating bread, pasta, potatoes, and cereals, opt for rice (preferably organic brown since it has not been stripped of valuable nutrients).

Keep dairy products to a minimum. Buy live, organic yogurt containing acidophilus and free of sugar or sugar substitutes.

Fact:

Bulgarian Yogurt is superior because it contains the most live cultures.

Olive oil is better than butter for cooking. Just don't overdo it! If you must have milk, be sure it is low-fat, skim, or soy, and try to limit your intake of cheese, particularly the aged cheeses.

In a recent study conducted at the University of California-Berkeley, researchers found that by eating every two to three hours instead of three big meals, the body's metabolism stays elevated and there is less chance of blood sugar levels fluctuating. Such fluctuation stimulates appetite and induces cravings. Eating smaller meals is beneficial to your digestive system and may also assist in a weight loss program.

This may seem like a lot; but as you read over the detoxifying tips, you will see that all we have really done is suggest nothing more than healthy eating habits. By incorporating these few things into your routine, you will feel better, be doing great things for your health, and, as a bonus, you will be staving off illness, even premature aging. Getting rid of toxins and unwanted waste is going to have an amazing effect on your overall well-being and your appearance.

Once your body has detoxified, and that is usually within a week or two, you may resume vigorous exercise (provided your physician says you are in good condition).

The detoxifying process we have described here is very conservative. There are many more specific detoxifying techniques and fasts you may want to explore once your body has adjusted to its new, healthier self.

> *Do not try any type of detoxification if you are pregnant, nursing, elderly, weak, or underweight.*

Fasting has been used for centuries to increase the process of elimination and the release of toxins from the colon, kidneys and bladder, lungs, sinuses, and skin. Fasting is helpful in clearing out the problems that have arisen from overeating and a sedentary lifestyle.

There are many different fasts, but the most popular are the juice fasts. Juice fasts include various forms of vegetable juices. Carrot, celery, green bean, parsley, watercress, and zucchini are among the most popular. Some people fast with vegetable broths, herbal teas, miso (fermented soy paste), and powdered algae. There is an excellent fast that suggests drinking a mixture of garlic, lemon juice, grapefruit juice, and olive oil at bedtime. (The combination is thought to detoxify the liver.) Juice fasts usually last around ten days. Since they are fairly long and restrictive, these fasts should not be undertaken too frequently. Done regularly, fasts can be very beneficial, but you should only attempt a fast if you are in good health.

> ***Ultimate Living Green Miracle*** *and* ***Aloe-Papaya Drink*** *offer wonderful added benefits during a fast.*

> *Avoid fasting if you have advanced cancer, heart problems, kidney disease, liver disease, diabetes, lung problems, or tuberculosis.*

Once you have cleansed your system, your body is better able to absorb nutrition and supplementation. Your immune system gets a rest from battling toxins and waste, and you should experience renewed energy and a sense of well-being.

Chapter Fourteen

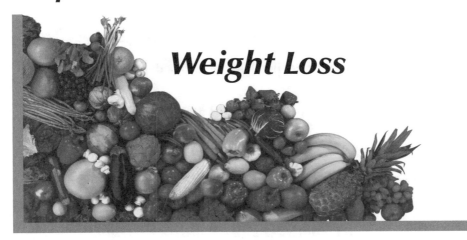

Weight Loss

Do you need good reasons to lose weight?

How about these:

- diabetes

- heart disease

- stroke

- hypertension

- gallbladder disease

- osteoarthritis (degeneration of cartilage and bone of joints)

- sleep apnea and other breathing problems

- some forms of cancer (uterine, breast, prostate, colorectal, kidney, and gallbladder)

- high blood cholesterol

- complications of pregnancy

- menstrual irregularities

- hirsutism (presence of excess body and facial hair)

- stress incontinence (urine leakage caused by weak pelvic-floor muscles)

- psychological disorders such as depression

- increased surgical risk

- decreased mental clarity

The United States Department of Health and Human Services provides the following statistics:

▷ Sixty-one percent of adults in the United States were overweight or obese (BMI > 25)* in 1999.

▷ Thirteen percent of children ages six to eleven years and fourteen percent of adolescents ages twelve to nineteen years were overweight in 1999. This prevalence has nearly tripled for adolescents in the past two decades.

▷ The increases in obesity and in those who are overweight cut across all ages, racial and ethnic groups, and both genders.

▷ Three hundred thousand deaths each year in the United States are associated with obesity.

▷ Being overweight and obesity are associated with heart disease, certain types of cancer, type 2 diabetes, stroke, arthritis, breathing problems, and psychological disorders such as depression.

▷ The economic cost of obesity in the United States was about $117 billion in 2000.

The following chart has done the calculations for you. Find your height in the left hand column and move to the right to find your weight. Your

BMI will be in the top line above where those two numbers intersect. If your BMI is 25 or over, you are in a higher risk for obesity-related illness. It is clear that obesity and being overweight are major health problems.

✳Body Mass Index

Body mass index, or BMI, is a new term to most people. However, it is the measurement of choice for many physicians and researchers studying obesity. BMI uses a mathematical formula that takes into account both a person's height and weight. BMI equals a person's weight in kilograms divided by height in meters squared (BMI=kg/m2).

BMI (kg/m²)	19	20	21	22	23	24	25	26	27	28	29	30	35	40
Height (in.)	Weight (lb.)													
58	91	96	100	105	110	115	119	124	129	134	138	143	167	191
59	94	99	104	109	114	119	124	128	133	138	143	148	173	198
60	97	102	107	112	118	123	128	133	138	143	148	153	179	204
61	100	106	111	116	122	127	132	137	143	148	153	158	185	211
62	104	109	115	120	126	131	136	142	147	153	158	164	191	218
63	107	113	118	124	130	135	141	146	152	158	163	169	197	225
64	110	116	122	128	134	140	145	151	157	163	169	174	204	232
65	114	120	126	132	138	144	150	156	162	168	174	180	210	240
66	118	124	130	136	142	148	155	161	167	173	179	186	216	247
67	121	127	134	140	146	153	159	166	172	178	185	191	223	255
68	125	131	138	144	151	158	164	171	177	184	190	197	230	262
69	128	135	142	149	155	162	169	176	182	189	196	203	236	270
70	132	139	146	153	160	167	174	181	188	195	202	207	243	278
71	136	143	150	157	165	172	179	186	193	200	208	215	250	286
72	140	147	154	162	169	177	184	191	199	206	213	221	258	294
73	144	151	159	166	174	182	189	197	204	212	219	227	265	302
74	148	155	163	171	179	186	194	202	210	218	225	233	272	311
75	152	160	168	176	184	192	200	208	216	224	232	240	279	319
76	156	164	172	180	189	197	205	213	221	230	238	246	287	328

Lose It!

Bad News—we are probably not telling you anything you don't already know—it is harder to lose weight as we age. In addition, besides putting us at risk for diseases, extra weight puts extra stress on our joints and bones and makes our heart work too hard.

Although weight loss has become a frenzied business–diets here, gyms everywhere–the best way to successfully take off those unwanted and unneeded pounds is to be realistic; set a good long-term goal; and start a healthy, low calorie, high fiber, and high nutrient diet plan. And, whatever else you do, **monitor your portions** and limit fats and sugars!

Some people feel they need special help to suppress their appetites. There are several good supplements on the market that will do so, but you must be very careful. There are many substances that can make you quite nervous or that may interact with other drugs that you might be taking.

> ***Ultimate Living Weight Loss*** *does not contain ma huang, ephedra, caffeine, or stimulants of any kind.*

Use It!

A healthy diet will help you lose weight; but if you combine your diet with exercise, the results will be much faster and you will feel that much better. You need regular aerobic exercise, exercise that boosts your heart rate, for at least thirty minutes three to four days a week. The beauty of walking is that it is something you can do today, requires little investment (a good pair of shoes), and it gets you out and about.

Find an activity you enjoy. You will not stick with a program unless you actually enjoy it. Try bicycling, hiking, horse-back riding, but find something you love to do. Vary your activities to avoid boredom and burnout.

The combination of weight-bearing and aerobic exercise plus a sensible eating plan will give you much better long-term results than "fad" diets.

Remember the Tin Man in The Wizard of Oz. He had been lying around for so long that all of his joints had frozen up. We can't rely on Dorothy, Toto, and the Scarecrow to get us up and moving. But before you jump up off the couch and jog to the next town, let's talk about the importance of warming up, stretching and limbering your body before exercise so you don't end up doing more harm than good. The more inactive you have been, the more important it is to start slowly, twenty or thirty minutes a day. It won't be long before you are able to do more.

It is important to remember to warm up and stretch before and after working out–even before walking. Warming up sends blood to the muscles and prepares them for activity, while stretching limbers your muscles, ligaments, and joints so you are far less apt to be sore and far less likely to receive an injury.

Exercise

The key to weight control is keeping energy intake (food) and energy output (physical activity) in balance. When you consume only as many calories as your body needs, your weight will usually remain constant. If you take in more calories than your body needs, you will put on excess fat. Exercise increases your energy output, calling on stored calories for extra fuel. Recent studies show that not only does exercise increase metabolism during a workout, but it also causes your metabolism to stay increased for a period of time after exercising, allowing you to burn more calories.

How much exercise is needed to make a difference in your weight depends on the amount of activity you perform and how much you eat. Aerobic exercise burns a combination of carbohydrates and stored body fat. You burn more fat with moderately intense exercise than with excessive cardiovascular activity. Remember, more time spent exercising does not necessarily mean more results. If you are walking, add some arm weights and vary the incline and speed of your walk. On a treadmill, you can adjust the incline and speed to enhance your results. For example, if you are walking at a pace of 3.8 mph, adjust up to 4.2 for two minutes and then down again. Do this every five or ten minutes.

You may want to increase the incline at lower speeds to build muscle and burn more fat. You will find that you will be able to exercise for shorter periods of time and see better results.

No matter what your age, you should incorporate some weight training into your exercise program. Muscle burns fat. The fastest way to gain results from exercising is to build lean muscle tissue. Strength training for as little as ten minutes per day or four times per week will help you to achieve your weight loss goals and put you one step closer to the body you desire.

It is best to perform aerobic exercise first thing in the morning or immediately after strength training for fat burning maximization. The reason for this is that it takes the body 20-30 minutes to start burning fat. After this period of time your muscles will release stored glycogen and begin to switch to a fat burning cycle. In the morning, your body does not have any glycogen or stored carbohydrates to burn. If you start your day by exercising, you will start your day burning fat.

If you consume 100 calories a day more than your body needs, you will gain about ten pounds in a year. You could take that weight off or keep it off by doing thirty minutes of moderate exercise daily. That's why experts agree that the key to weight control is a combination of exercise and diet.

Exercise is also known as physical activity and includes anything that gets you moving, such as walking, dancing, or working in the yard. You can earn the benefits of being physically active without going to a gym, playing sports, or using fancy equipment. When you're physically fit, you have the strength, flexibility, and endurance needed for your daily activities.

When starting an exercise program, find out which activities will be safe for you. Think about what activities are realistic and choose the ones you think you can do.

Then follow these guidelines:

- Start slowly. Your activity should be somewhat challenging but not overly difficult.

- Always do some simple stretching before and after any physical activity.

- Drink plenty of water before, during, and after activity.

- Keep a journal of your progress.

- Don't be too hard on yourself. If you don't feel like exercising, it may be that your body is trying to tell you something. Do something relaxing instead. Try deep breathing or some easy yoga positions.

Being physically active helps you feel better physically and mentally. You will find that the more you do, the more you will be capable of doing.

Stress and Weight Loss

Besides looking and feeling younger and definitely feeling better, exercise will help you De-Stress! Stress melts away when you are engaged in activities you truly enjoy. The benefit is that you will see pounds melting away as well.

Researchers now know that stress can inhibit weight loss. Stress releases certain hormones and chemicals into our systems that cause us to "hold on" to fat. The hormones released when we're stressed include adrenalin—which gives us instant energy—along with corticotrophin releasing hormone (CRH) and cortisol.

Cortisol is part of the "fight or flight" mechanism in our body that enabled our ancestors to run from saber-toothed tigers. Their adrenal glands would send cortisol into their bodies to give them the rush of energy they needed to escape. Our "saber-toothed tigers" are everyday stresses, and cortisol is still at work.

Excess cortisol can lead not only to weight gain but also to the tendency to store what is called "visceral fat" around the midsection. When you are under stress, cortisol tells your body to store fat for energy, and it especially encourages fat deposits around the abdomen. These fat cells that lie deep within the abdomen have been linked to an increase in both diabetes and heart disease.

Part of the problem is that you are more likely to have cravings when you are under stress. In other words, since your neuro-endocrine system doesn't know you didn't fight or flee, it still responds to stress with the hormonal signal to replenish nutritional stores—which may make you feel hungry. The so-called comfort foods (starchy and fat foods) stimulate the production of seratonin, a feel-good chemical in the body. When such cravings occur, instead of reaching for cookies and cake, reach for lean turkey, bananas, or other similar foods that raise seratonin levels.

> ***Ultimate Living Green Miracle*** *will take away cravings for comfort food.*

At the same time, stress inhibits your digestive system. Stress frequently causes digestive and bowel discomforts such as diarrhea and constipation. When you are not eliminating properly, wastes and toxins are allowed to build up in your system. Your body no longer burns fat or performs efficiently.

Now for the good news—whether your urge to eat is driven by hormones or habits or a combination of both, research shows there are ways to interrupt the cycle, break the stress, and stop the weight gain.

Here's what the experts recommend:

▷ **Exercise.** This is the best stress buster—and it also happens to be good for you in lots of other ways.

▷ **Eat a balanced diet—and do not allow yourself to become hungry. Do not skip meals.** This helps keep blood sugar levels steady, and this in turn puts a damper on insulin production and eventually reduces cortisol levels—all helping to control appetite and weight.

▷ **Don't lose sleep.** When we don't get enough rest, cortisol levels rise.

▷ **Devote time to relaxation**—Relaxing works much like exercise to produce brain chemicals that counter the effects of stress.

▷ **Snack on whole grain, high fiber foods.** If you just can't ignore those stress-related hunger pangs, try foods high in fiber and low in sugar such as oatmeal, whole-wheat bread, or fruits such as pears or plums.

▷ **Avoid caffeine, cigarettes, and alcohol**—According to the American Institute of Stress, cigarettes, as well as caffeine-laden soft drinks, coffee, tea, and even chocolate, can cause cortisol levels to rise, stress to increase, blood sugar to drop, and hunger to prevail. The institute also cautions against drinking too much alcohol, which can affect blood sugar and insulin levels.

➢ **Take your vitamins**—A number of medical studies have shown that stress can deplete important nutrients—particularly the B complex and C vitamins and sometimes the minerals calcium and magnesium. These nutrients are needed to balance the effects of stress hormones such as cortisol and may even play a role in helping us burn fat.

> Taking a high potency multi-vitamin supplement such as **Ultimate Living Multi-Vitamin** can insure you give your body what it needs not only to deal with the stress but also to burn fat and lose weight.

Eating Less–The Hardest Part

We are blessed to live in a country with plenty of food. But plenty should not mean super-sized. Restaurant portions are entirely too large. Portion control is essential in a successful weight loss program.

The American Institute for Cancer Research (AICR) notes that obesity became an epidemic in America at the same time that portion size grew. The food industry's "value marketing" strategy of offering more for less has also affected Americans' waistlines as well as their wallets. "It's not what you eat but how much you eat that counts most when it comes to weight reduction," says Melanie Polk, director for nutrition education at AICR.

To help Americans slim down and eat healthier, the AICR has created a new approach to eating called "The New American Plate." Very simply, it advises people to focus on portion size when making meals at home or ordering out at restaurants.

What should be on the new American plate? Nutritionists agree that vegetables, fruits, whole grains, and beans should cover two-thirds or more of the plate. Meats and other animal-source foods should cover one-third or less. Research has shown that fruits and vegetables have a protective effect against cancer because of the phytochemicals they contain. Phytochemicals interfere with cancer cell growth and reproduction.

The new American plate is almost a reversal of the old American plate, which typically featured eight to ten ounces of steak with buttery mashed potatoes and peas. Where's the beef under the new plan? People are urged to think of meat as a side dish or condiment rather than the primary ingredient.

U.S. Department of Agriculture statistics show that the average daily caloric intake of Americans has risen from 1,854 calories to 2,002 calories during the last twenty years. That increase–148 calories per day–theoretically works out to an extra fifteen pounds per year.

Practice portion control

Here are some tips for adjusting to portion control:

> **Use the "eyeball method":** Fill a measuring cup or spoon with a single serving of a favorite food (the precise amount is found on the "Nutrition Facts" label) and empty it onto a clean plate or bowl. By "eyeballing" the plate or bowl, you can get a sense of what single servings look like. Polk says many people will be surprised to learn that the bowl of cereal they eat every morning contains twice or even three times more servings (and fat and calories and sugar) than they realize.

> **Make substitutions.** Choose a regular burger instead of the quarter-pounder for a saving of 160 calories. Use sunflower seeds instead of a handful of greasy croutons on your salad, and use low-fat milk on your cereal.

> **Think small; divide in half and share.** If you're given the option when dining out, order half an entree or order small—a cup of soup instead of a bowl, for example, or an appetizer and soup instead of an entree. Also, ask for an order to be divided between two people. "You have to let them know there's too much food on that plate," Polk says.

> **Doggie-bagging dinner.** At table-service restaurants, ask the server to put half of your entree in a doggie bag before bringing it to your table. This strategy, says Polk, is not only calorie effective, but it provides two full meals for the price of one.

*Many of us eat when we are happy, sad, or nervous. Emotions can affect your appetite, but here are some overeating triggers that may surprise you (from "Beat Overeating Triggers," Cooking Light Magazine, **November, 2002**).*

> **Dim lighting:** The dimmer the lighting, the higher the likelihood of overindulgence, says a study from the University of California at Irvine. Why? "Brighter lighting forces you to be more aware of what you're eating," says Joe Kasof, Ph.D., lead study author. **Beat it by:** Sitting outdoors or near windows, using brighter bulbs in your lamps, adding lighting to eating areas, or moving to a brighter room.

> **Distractions:** In another study, when women who normally watched what they ate listened to a taped detective story, they consumed more calories. Researchers suspect the story interfered with the women's focus on keeping calories in check. **Beat it by:** Clearing all distractions; let the enjoyment of the meal provide your focus.

▷ **Low energy:** "When your energy's low, you may look for food to pick you up," says Robert E. Thayer, Ph.D., professor of psychology at California State University at Long Beach. Unfortunately, most people reach for calorie-laden treats instead of an apple or banana.

Beat it by: Identifying your low-energy times of day and substituting other activities for eating. Take a ten minute walk or a water-cooler chat break.

Be a label reader

It's a well known fact that over consumption of foods high in fat and calories causes weight gain. Instead of eliminating all your favorite fattening foods, try reducing their fat and calorie content. When making a food choice, choose those low in fat and calories and nutrient rich in vitamins and minerals. Some foods supply empty calories, providing most of their calories from sugar and fat and giving you few if any vitamins and minerals. When you are grocery shopping, always read the food labels to find out the calorie and fat contents.

Remember that many foods that are listed as low-fat are very high in calories. Also, natural foods such as vegetables, fruits, and whole grains are naturally low in fat.

When grocery shopping, shop the perimeter of the store. The outer perimeter contains produce, protein, and dairy. Stay away from pre-packaged, processed, and frozen foods that can be loaded with hidden preservatives, colorings, and fat.

Tips for Success

People fail at weight loss for any number of reasons, but there are a few things you can do to increase your chances for success.

> **Set The Right Goals.** Setting the right goals is an important first step. Make your goals attainable, realistic, and specific. For instance, rather than deciding to exercise more, decide to walk 45 minutes a day. A specific, attainable goal will give you a feeling of achievement and success.

> **Allow yourself to be successful.** Rather than a weight loss goal of two pounds a week, make your goal three pounds a month, and you will not get frustrated staring at the scales. Instead, after that first successful month, you will realize that weight loss is attainable.

> **Recognize the pitfalls.** If you are inclined to snack while you watch television, go out and take a walk instead of parking yourself in the chair. If there are friends who encourage you to eat too much, you need to socialize with them in situations that do not involve food.

> **Know when to stop!** Most people eat beyond that feeling of fullness. Learn to eat slowly and stop when you begin to feel full. You will find that within a very few minutes you are satisfied.

Fad diets abound. The book shelves are brimming with the latest "new" ways to lose weight. In truth, there is only one way to lose weight and that is to eat less and exercise more. By losing weight in a sensible, healthy manner, you will not only be improving your appearance, but more importantly, you will be adding good healthy years to your life.

Remember! Obesity is more than a cosmetic problem; it's a health hazard!

Chapter Fifteen

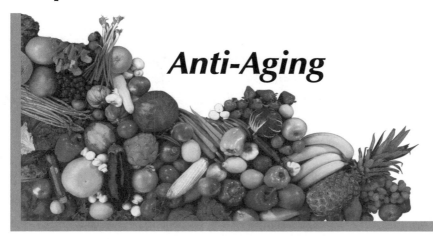

Anti-Aging

In 2004, American consumers spent almost $45 billion on anti-aging products and services, and the total anti-aging market is projected to reach over $70 billion by 2009. Clearly we are trying to remain feeling and looking young.

In the 1950's, women (and men) began having "face-lifts" and, with the possible exception of Jack Lalane, did not worry too much about the physiological aspects of aging. These days people not only want to look younger, but they also want to remain feeling young too. We now know that remaining physically younger is possible, mainly by staving off premature aging.

The same factors that lead to disease also lead to aging. While it is true that each of us knows someone in his or her nineties who smoked all his or her life and spent the last half century of life watching television, most octogenarians share one thing–an active lifestyle. Living longer seems to include plenty of physical activity, nutritious foods, being able to relax and enjoy life, and an involvement in one's community.

The first and foremost way to stave off aging is to stay healthy. We have already discussed the importance of keeping your immune system in top shape to ward off disease, but it is, in fact, your immune system that plays the greatest role in aging.

Nutrition for Anti-Aging

Research suggests that those same antioxidants that bolster your immune system can keep you looking and feeling young. This means a diet loaded with antioxidant-rich fruits and vegetables and supplementation to increase your antioxidant levels.

We have already talked about free radicals, but those little "energy vampires" can also sap your body's and skin's youthful feeling and appearance. Our own bodies generate free radicals as by-products of exercising, fighting infection, and even breathing. In these processes some of our oxygen molecules lose an electron. These molecules are now free radicals, and they are desperate to become stable. Consequently, they attach themselves to whatever they contact. This process is known as oxidative damage, and it is the underlying factor of many chronic illnesses and aging. Antioxidants are our salvation against free radicals.

Things such as stress and air pollution produce free radicals and therefore gobble up our stores of antioxidants. The body has its own army of antioxidants. Our "army," however, needs reinforcements, and we obtain them through diet and supplementation.

Pollution, exposure to toxic substances in the environment, and stress are all triggers for free radicals. Most Americans live in urban environments where these factors are unavoidable. To combat these occurrences, we must insure that our bodies receive enough antioxidants from our diets and a good program of supplementation.

Vitamin C

Vitamin C remains the general in the army of antioxidants. Studies have shown vitamin C to cut the risk of many cancers and to help lower the risk of cardiovascular disease. Vitamin C also seems to have a neutralizing effect on certain carcinogenic (cancer-causing) agents such as nitrites used in curing meats and cigarette smoking. The greater the oxidative stress, the more antioxidants a person must ingest through diet or supplementation. For example, people who smoke need three times more vitamin C than non-smokers.

Vitamin C occurs abundantly in nature in fruits and vegetables, particularly citrus fruits, berries, tomatoes, green leafy vegetables, and the cabbages.

> ***Ultimate Living Green Miracle*** and ***Aloe-Papaya Drink*** are *loaded with vitamin C.*

Salads are an important part of a healthy diet. A salad can be a starter or a meal in itself. In preparing salads you just need imagination in combining variations of vegetables, fruits, herbs, and other healthy components. Salads are a great way to obtain valuable antioxidants.

Vitamin E

Of the eight forms of vitamin E that occur in nature, it appears that alpha-tocopherol is the main defense against the oxidation of lipids (fats). Vitamin E also helps break free radical chain reactions. Vitamin C is water soluble, but vitamin E is fat soluble, therefore acting within cell membranes and other fat-containing tissues.

Research suggests that vitamin E protects against heart disease and stroke. It also seems to have positive effects on immunity in the elderly. Vitamin E may protect cells from the cancerous effects of x-rays, chemicals, air pollutants, and ultraviolet light. Insufficient intake of vitamin E correlates with an increased risk of lung, colon, stomach, breast, and cervical cancer.

Sources of vitamin E are oils, nuts, and grains–all high in fat. Supplements are a good source of vitamin E without the calories.

Ultimate Living Multi-Vitamin contains 400 IU of pure vitamin E.

CoQ10

Coenzyme Q10 (CoQ10) has the potential to improve energy production in mitochondria (parts of a cell where aerobic production takes place). CoQ10 is necessary for human life to exist, and a deficiency can contribute to ill health and disease. It also helps prevent and treat various diseases and conditions. It is a proven treatment for cardiovascular diseases, hypertension, periodontal disease, stomach ulcers, and impotence. It also aids in weight loss and improves aerobic performance. It is known to be an energy booster and immune system enhancer.

CoQ10 is made in the body and occurs naturally in all cells; but as we get older, its production falls. CoQ10 can also be found in food but in very small amounts. This is why it is very important to take CoQ10 supplements.

Minerals

Our bodies can manufacture vitamins but not minerals. We must obtain minerals from our diets or from supplements.

All minerals are antioxidants. Selenium, zinc, copper, manganese, and iron are all components of antioxidant enzymes.

Selenium has been the most widely studied mineral and has been shown to retard cancers in both animal and human studies. Selenium occurs naturally in many plants, including garlic, asparagus, and grains.

Today's farming practices have almost completely stripped our top soils of minerals and have left our foods depleted of vital nutrition. Coupled with the fact that our foods are sprayed with chemical toxins and are bleached, processed, and synthetically preserved, we are left with foods that are a shadow of their former selves fifty plus years ago. Vitamins are a necessary and vital part of our health but simply cannot work without proper mineral supplementation to create the synergy needed for the vitamins to be absorbed.

Ultimate Living Ionic Trace Minerals are the most readily absorbable minerals available. To be assimilated in the body, minerals need to enter in the ionic form. Colloidal minerals are ground up rocks with a molecular structure too large to penetrate the cell walls. Even when they are suspended in liquid, the body must break down the colloidal minerals into an ionic form, which compromises the ability of the mineral to penetrate the cell wall. Ionic minerals, on the other hand, enter through the cell wall immediately because they are already broken down into their smallest molecular structure. They are in a true solution and are capable of being directly absorbed into the bloodstream. Ionic minerals are actually pure, living minerals that conduct and produce electrical energies to keep living things alive and allow cellular regeneration and healing.

Ultimate Living Ionic Trace Minerals come from the Great Salt Lake. These ionic minerals are the most concentrated minerals available—26 times more concentrated than colloidal minerals, and they provide over 50 minerals in nature's perfect balance. The Great Salt Lake is a miracle of Mother Nature. It has been concentrating mineral salts in its waters for thousands of years. Not only is it the world's richest source of liquid ionic minerals and trace minerals, but it is also one of the finest purification plants ever created. The total soluble concentrations of heavy metals in the water are extremely low. The natural heat of the sun precipitates the sediments and any alien matter. The lake thus avoids any accumulation of heavy metals and is nontoxic and self-cleansing.

Our bodies are marvelous electrical machines, and minerals are necessary to orchestrate a symphony of complete harmony within our cells. **Ultimate Living Ionic Trace Minerals** *are powerful conductors of this electrical activity. Ionic trace minerals work like "nature's sparkplugs" in activating the vitamins and nutrients in our bodies. Some symptoms of mineral deficiency are prolonged wound healing, loss of taste, increase in sugar cravings, beginnings of osteoporosis, painful joints, lack of energy, rapid pulse, and nervousness, to name a few.*

If you are feeling fatigued or you are wondering why you are not getting a burst of energy from your daily intake of vitamins and organic foods, you are most likely mineral deficient. In order to get the most out of your daily regimen, be sure to include **Ultimate Living Ionic Trace Minerals** *and start reaping the benefits of optimum health.*

Phytochemicals

Phytochemicals in plants protect against free radical damage, LDL cholesterol oxidation, blood vessel fragility, dementia, macular degeneration, and cancer. Carotenoids and flavonoids are two groups of phytochemicals that have been shown to have anti-aging properties.

Carotenoids are potent phytochemicals abundant in yellow, orange, red, and green fruits and vegetables.

The best known carotenoid is beta-carotene which seems to have a neutralizing influence on the damage to the skin, eyes, and lungs caused by air pollution and the sun.

Another valuable carotenoid is lycopene, the red pigment abundant in tomatoes. Lycopene is ten times more powerful than beta-carotene. Research suggests that lycopene protects men against prostate cancer. Lutein and zeaxanthin, abundant in spinach, are recommended to protect the eyes from macular degeneration, a disease of aging that eventually causes loss of sight.

Flavonoids

Flavonoids form the water-soluble colors of vegetables, fruit, grain, seeds, leaves, and bark. Grapes, and the juices and wines made from them, are rich in flavonoids called catechins. Red grapes and their products contain an additional antioxidant, anthocyanin, that gives them their intense red-purple color. Green and black teas contain large amounts of catechin flavonoids.

The French who consume large quantities of wine have a relatively low incident of heart disease. It is thought that the flavonoids in red wine may have artery-cleansing effects.

The onion family—garlic, onions, shallots, and leeks—contains flavonoids, vitamin C, selenium, and sulfur-containing substances.

Cruciferous vegetables, vegetables such as cabbage, broccoli, and brussel sprouts, have antioxidant capabilities because of their high vitamin C and flavonoid content. They also contain plant chemicals that help to neutralize carcinogens.

Isoflavones

Isoflavones are a type of flavonoid that has weak estrogenic activity and can compete with the body's own estrogen. This may be part of the reason the Japanese, who eat a diet low in fat and rich in soy and green tea, have low rates of breast, prostate, and colorectal cancer.

Ginkgo tree leaf extracts

Ginkgo tree leaf extracts are thought to improve brain function. For centuries, Chinese medicine has focused on the health properties of ginkgo.

Free radical damage is cumulative with age. People should start supplementing with antioxidants early to achieve long-term benefits. Antioxidants are powerful weapons in the war against aging. By combating free radical induced damage, we may be able to live longer and have healthier lives!

B vitamins

B vitamins are essential for good health and longevity.

> *Increased homocysteine levels in the body not only increase a person's risk of heart attack (Chapter Three) by 300 percent. Increased homocysteine levels are also partially responsible for many diseases and symptoms associated with aging such as lack of energy, memory loss, heart disease, stroke, bone fractures, shingles, anemia, Alzheimer's disease, and dementia.*
>
> *The combination of vitamins B-6, B-12, and folic acid can be very effective in helping to lower homocysteine levels.*

Vitamin B-6 is involved in more body functions than almost any other single nutrient. It is needed for the metabolism of proteins, helps to maintain fluid balance, and is required for healthy red blood cells. It can be found in seaweed, liver, meat, and fish.

Vitamin B-12 is needed for the production of red blood cells and the maintenance of the protective sheath around nerves. It is found in oysters, salmon, mackerel, herring, and seaweed.

Folic acid is needed for energy production and protein metabolism. It regulates the formation of red blood cells and aids in the proper formation and functioning of white blood cells. It prevents anemia, helps with depression and anxiety, and also helps you sleep. (Folic acid is very important for pregnant women to sustain pregnancy and prevent birth defects.)

Ultimate Living B Complex-Lingual is a powerful combination of all three B vitamins to be placed under the tongue where it is easily assimilated by the body. The B-12 methylcobalamin in Ultimate Living B Complex-Lingual is the most bioavailable form of the nutrient with 98 percent absorption when taken sublingually (under the tongue)–the same absorption rate as an injection but less painful. If you are experiencing symptoms of aging, try Ultimate Living B Complex-Lingual and help yourself experience a rejuvenation.

Lifestyle and Anti-Aging

Low Fat–Low Calorie

Being overweight, particularly being obese, contributes to any number of debilitating diseases from arthritis to cancer and diabetes.

Diet is a critical factor in anti-aging. You need to eliminate saturated fats and excess protein that create toxicity in the body, especially the liver, all the while making us feel fatigued.

Carbohydrates are best obtained from whole grains, fruits, and vegetables rather than from white breads, pastas, cakes, and desserts.

Eating smaller meals is easier on the digestive system and maintains a better balance of glucose levels.

It is never too late to begin to pay attention to the nutritional value of the foods you are consuming, and in so doing, you will automatically lose weight and be able to effortlessly maintain your ideal body weight.

Hydration

Pure drinking water helps to hydrate the body and keep the cells young. Make sure that you are drinking pure water, not tap water loaded with chemicals that tax the immune system. The best water has been through the reverse osmosis process. Carry a bottle of water with you and sip it consistently, especially when engaged in physical activity. Thirst is your body's way of saying that it is dehydrated, and dehydration is hard on all of your organs, especially your skin.

Drinking plenty of water not only keeps the body hydrated, but it also helps in the elimination of toxins.

Fasting

Fasting is a great way to detoxify the body and give the immune system a rest. Fasting has its foundation in religious practices. It is actually a holy tradition. The apostles fasted, and they knew that gluttony was a sin.

Fasting does not have to be too difficult. Following a fast, you should feel re-energized and have a brighter mental outlook. (See chapter 13, page 237)

The Environment

We have already discussed pollution and stress, but it should be emphasized that these two factors together with disease tax the body's stores of vital nutrients more than any others. In order to remain feeling and looking younger, we need to assess our lifestyles and make appropriate changes today.

Your Environment

Your immediate surroundings play a role in your overall health. It is important that your home be as clean as possible. Indoor air pollution can be as harmful as outdoor. If you suffer from allergies, the importance of keeping your environment free of dust and animal dander is crucial.

Invest in a good HEPA (High Efficiency Particulate Air) filter.

Physical Activity

Moderate exercise can significantly improve one's health and longevity. Exercise does the following:

- relieves stress, lowers blood pressure, and increases the level of endorphins (brain hormones that increase the feeling of happiness and well-being)

- speeds up the fat burning enzymes in the muscles and helps you stay fit and maintain weight loss

- strengthens heart muscles and improves circulation of blood, reducing the risk of heart disease

- reduces the level of glucose and cholesterol in the blood

- improves your respiratory system, strengthens your lungs, and helps to control asthma

- creates the feeling of self-confidence and a sense of control over one's body and life

Mainly due to all these benefits of moderate exercise, physical activity is considered to be essential for those who want to lengthen their life span.

Rest and Relaxation

The link between "life-quality" and longevity is widely accepted. You should create a place within your environment to escape everyday tensions and stresses. Even a person living in a city apartment can create a special place to experience pleasant memories and images. A garden area, a porch, or a balcony can be a great place to sit and reflect. Making your own special place provides a sense of security and "home." If you are a bird lover, buy a feeder. If you love plants, surround yourself with flowers. Most people respond to the sound of water. Fountains are great "relaxers," and with today's mini-fountains, anyone can find a space.

We're born knowing how to relax. As infants we instinctively relax and sleep when our bodies and minds need a break. As we age, we control our urges to sleep or relax since we must remain alert as we go about our life duties. We often spend years working and performing beyond exhaustion. Consequently, when we have an opportunity to relax, we are conditioned not to do so.

Relaxation is individual. Physical activity may relax one person, while sitting down reading a book may relax another. Some people need structure such as meditation or yoga. Whatever your preference, take time daily to practice relaxation. It will add years to your life.

Many of us do not even realize that we are not relaxing. Even at rest, we breathe shallow breaths and have tensed muscles. You need to practice relaxation techniques for at least twenty to thirty minutes per day, and it would be beneficial to learn some technique that puts you in a relaxed state. Meditation is ideal.

A variation of the meditation technique known as the relaxation response has gained popularity in the U.S. since its description in the 1970s by Harvard physician Herbert Benson. This technique involves the repetition of a word or phrase while being quietly seated, ten to twenty minutes per day. Its value has been documented in the reduction of blood pressure and other bodily stress responses. The relaxation response requires practice, but the effort is well worth it.

Staying Involved

For decades research has shown a link between having a good quality of life and having meaningful relationships with other people. Science documents the effects of social support systems on one's health. A growing body of evidence suggests that maintaining relationships can reduce some of the health-related impacts of aging. Now the thinking is that relationships and interaction with others may add to your longevity.

Staying involved with your community can mean different things to different people. Becoming older means you have more time, plenty of wisdom, and experience to share. Put those assets to work by offering your time and talents. Tutor at an elementary school, work at a food bank, campaign for a favorite political candidate, or deliver for Meals on Wheels. Volunteer with an organization whose cause you support; or head to your local library, a church, or a religious group to find out about more volunteer opportunities.

Family ties, friendships, and involvement in social activities can offer a psychological buffer against stress, anxiety, and depression. Social support can both help protect you against developing an illness and assist you in coping better with medical problems. It may even increase your life span.

Some ideas to increase your social interaction:

- Pets are great ice-breakers. If you don't have a dog, get one. Having a pet increases your longevity too, especially if you get out and walk.

- Join a class through a local gym, senior center, or community fitness facility. Or start a lunchtime walking group at work.

- Hospitals, churches, museums, community centers, and other organizations often need volunteers. You can form strong connections when you work with people with a mutual goal.

- Get together with a group of people working toward a goal you believe in such as an election or the cleanup of a natural area.

- Find a nearby group with similar interests in such things as auto racing, music, gardening, books, or crafts.

- Take a college or community education course to meet people with similar interests. Exercising your mind keeps you young.

It seems that everyone is in search of a magic bullet for anti-aging. There is no one guarantee for youth, but following the suggestions in this chapter will insure your feeling better and younger and may well allow you to feel better and look younger longer.

Chapter Sixteen

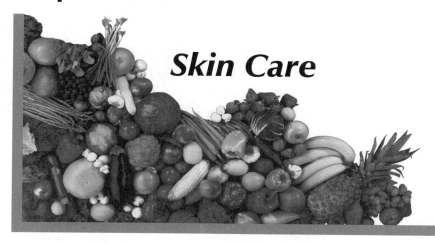

Skin Care

I If you do not want to look old, then you are never too young to start a good skin care regimen.

As the largest organ, skin serves several functions. Besides being a protective covering for our internal systems and organs, skin is part of our respiratory system. Toxins are eliminated through the skin in the form of perspiration.

Many skin conditions may be a direct reflection of our environment, genetics, diet, how much water we drink, hormones, or even how much sleep we receive.

> **Environment:** Recent studies show that approximately 80 percent of premature aging is actually the result of sun damage that could have been prevented. The ultraviolet rays penetrate through the epidermis and the dermis to destroy our valuable connective tissue. Our skin should always be protected from the sun as overexposure can lead to premature aging, wrinkles, dryness, and possibly skin cancer.

▷ **Diet:** If we are not getting the right nourishment, our skin cell production and rejuvenating properties will suffer. Green foods provide an excellent source of antioxidant protection, helping to prevent cellular damage that leads to skin degradation. Proper nutrition enables our body to function properly in healing, restoring, and strengthening all cells. To combat signs of premature aging, be sure your diet includes plenty of fresh vegetables and fruits along with proper supplements.

Ultimate Living Green Miracle provides antioxidant protection as well as all of your required servings of organic fruits and vegetables.

▷ **Water:** Drink as much water as possible; water is an excellent balancer for the skin. Try to drink at a minimum eight to ten glasses daily. To insure you are receiving the proper amount of water, take your body weight and divide in half. Yes, you read it right! This is the number of ounces of water you should be drinking daily. If you have noticed darkness under your eyes, this is often because the skin is dehydrated. You need more water in your system.

If you are a caffeine drinker, drink two glasses of water for every cup of coffee you consume to avoid dehydration.

▷ **Hormones:** Certainly wrinkles may be caused by any number of things. One possible cause of wrinkles could be hormone imbalance. Proper hormone levels are essential for healthy living. Healthy living for women means strong bones, healthy hearts, and freedom from major menopausal symptoms. A change in hormone levels plays a major role in the appearance of our skin. During puberty young girls may experience acne; during pregnancy a woman may develop dry, red facial patches; and during menopause you will see a definite change in your skin. Remember, anything that takes place internally is reflected externally. When there is a hormone imbalance, skin cell reproduction slows down; so collagen and elastin cells diminish, leading to wrinkles, fine lines, and saggy skin.

➢ **Sleep** is one of the necessities of life. It is as important as food, water, and proper nutrition. Sleep is a restorative process that replenishes the nerve energy needed for many body processes. It is during this time that the body renews itself, ridding the system of toxins. Studies have shown that body cells heal, strengthen, and rebuild while we sleep.

We believe the body requires eight hours of sleep each night.

The harsh, drying effects of the sun, time, and the environment may rob our skin of the vital nutrients and essential moisture needed to maintain a youthful glow. Good skin care maintenance begins with both internal and external strategies. A combination of a healthy lifestyle, a good nutritional program, and a home care routine from head to toe will strengthen, nourish, and protect our skin.

Healthy-looking skin is one of our most valuable assets. Appearance is an important psychological factor for young and old alike. Clear, beautiful, youthful skin is not only attractive, but it makes you look and feel great. It can build self-confidence and self-esteem.

Nutrition for the Skin

To maintain health and wellness, we already know how important it is to include a rich source of vitamins, minerals, and antioxidants in our daily diet. It is just as important to ensure that the outside of our body, the skin, is nourished and protected with those same nutrients.

Vitamins for the Inside

Taken internally these nutrients have positive effects on skin health and appearance.

A good multivitamin is the foundation of a good supplement program. Your multi-vitamin should provide you with basic nutrition and should act as a foundation for your supplement program.

> *Ultimate Living Multi-Vitamin contains all the essential ingredients for maximum protection.*

Antioxidants–Vitamins A, C, E, and grape seed extract have excellent anti-aging properties. Free radicals are almost solely responsible for skin's aging. Antioxidants fight free radicals and can lead the charge in the battle against time.

> *Ultimate Living Super Antioxidant is fifty times more potent than vitamin C and 20 times more potent than vitamin E.*

Vitamin A can be found in eggs, brightly colored fruits and vegetables, fish liver oil, dairy products, beef, liver, milk, carrots, and tomatoes.

Vitamin C is abundant in tomatoes, cherries, broccoli, strawberries, and chilies. The oxidation process that causes skin damage, including discolorations and wrinkling from free radicals, is greatly reduced by vitamin C in skin care formulations.

Vitamin E can be found in cold pressed oils, whole wheat, sweet potatoes, molasses, nuts, dark green vegetables, eggs, oatmeal, and wheat germ. Vitamin E is absolutely known to smooth the skin and increase its moisture content. It is now thought that vitamin E may reduce wrinkles and that it may even prevent collagen loss from free radical damage.

Grape seed extract contains proanthocyanidins that are 20 times more potent than vitamin C and 50 times more potent than vitamin E. They are found in the peel of fruits and vegetables as well as the bark of some trees such as lemon trees.

Essential fatty acids (EFA's)–Many types of skin disorders such as eczema and psoriasis can be cleared within weeks based on a regimen that incorporates generous essential fatty acids. They are great for your heart and may offer cancer protection as well. Skin cells will better absorb moisturizers and treatments with the help of EFA's. Try getting your EFA's for your skin from flax oil.

Calcium–Calcium is best absorbed when accompanied by other minerals such as magnesium and vitamin D. Calcium helps to strengthen the structure that makes up your countenance–bone structure. Plus, calcium gives you strong, beautiful nails.

> *Ultimate Living Cal-Mag provides the perfect balance of calcium, magnesium and vitamin D.*

Green foods are full of antioxidants to fight free radicals–skin's enemies– and they contribute to overall health, therefore overall appearance.

> *Ultimate Living Green Miracle, full of live green foods, is a great source of antioxidants.*

B vitamins–B vitamin deficiencies can cause tough, dry skin. B vitamins are in whole grains, liver, brewer's yeast, nuts, wheat germ, poultry, brown rice, egg yolks, legumes, blackstrap molasses, whole wheat, potatoes, cheese, milk, yogurt, cantaloupe, meat, peas, leafy green vegetables, prunes, soy beans, lentils, oats, root vegetables, sardines, tuna, and salmon.

> *Two **Ultimate Living B-Complex Lingual** tablets daily deliver all the required B-vitamin needs as well as the perfect amount of folic acid.*

Minerals enable the body to properly assimilate all other nutrients.

> ***Ultimate Living Ionic Trace Minerals** are a formulation of the only minerals small enough to actually penetrate the body's cellular structure.*

Enzymes help the body properly eliminate toxins that can cause the skin to look dull and sallow.

> ***Ultimate Living Complete Enzymes** are effective in promoting digestive health to improve skin texture, clarity, and appearance.*

Vitamins for the Outside *(on the skin)*

When applied to the skin, these substances increase its moisture and vitality:

> ▷ **Hyaluronic acid,** a key component of collagen, has been called a "space filler" or "support scaffolding" for living cells. It makes up much of the material in between cells and provides structure to various organs such as the eyes, joints, and skin. Hyaluronic acid is akin to mortar in a brick wall. It holds the cells in place. Hyaluronic acid, however, breaks down and is produced less as we age. Collagen degradation accounts for most of the overt signs of

aging in the human body. Applied topically, hyaluronic acid grabs moisture and holds it, hydrating cells and smoothing the skin.

▷ **Alpha lipoic acid** is a strong antioxidant excellent for skin health. This anti-aging antioxidant repairs, heals, and stimulates skin cells. Use of alpha lipoic acid on the skin may help to promote and develop a supple, youthful, and glowing appearance. Its use has been tested and been shown to reduce wrinkles and pore size while producing a clearer, healthier looking complexion.

▷ **Aloe vera** is known as the "healing plant." The gel of the aloe vera has been used for centuries to treat cuts and burns. It is a soothing salve for irritations and redness.

▷ **Green tea** isn't just to drink. When applied to the skin it causes skin cells to rebuild and redevelop. Green tea helps make new skin.

▷ **Arnica** is an anti-inflammatory that reduces puffiness and bruising.

▷ **Eyebright extract** reduces puffiness and feeds cell skin structure.

▷ **Vitamin E** is a natural skin protectant.

Diet

Vegetables and Fruits—We believe you cannot get enough vegetables and fruits in your diet. The more color in fruits and vegetables, the more antioxidants. Learn to eat your fruits and veggies in as near a natural state as possible. We also recommend buying organic whenever possible. Of course fresh and raw is best, but lightly steamed is fine, too. That way your body receives everything that veggies and fruits have to offer, and they offer our bodies a great deal—protection from disease, help for our immune systems, and, once again, protection from free radicals through their antioxidants properties. That is where vegetables and fruits come in to help our skin stay younger, fresher, and healthier looking.

Remember! Three scoops of **Ultimate Living Green Miracle** give you the equivalent of one and one half pounds of organic fruits and vegetables.

Essential nutrition for skin includes the following:

➤ **Protein** is essential in our bodies' building blocks. The body cannot heal itself without protein. Cancer patients are told to eat plenty of protein for this exact reason. This does not mean you should sit down to a sixteen ounce sirloin at every meal; but you should include eggs, plenty of cold water fish (especially salmon), poultry, beans, and some beef in your everyday diet.

➤ **Whole grains**–Our ancestors very nearly existed on whole grains, and you need them too. When people refer to bread as the "staff of life," they are not referring to plastic-bagged white bread. If you eat bread, it should be wholesome 100 percent whole wheat or whole grain. Sprouted grain is best. Breads can be good for you but not white, refined, sugar-loaded breads. Find a healthy bakery (there may be one within your own grocery store) and learn to enjoy whole grain breads with pure-fruit jams.

➤ **Fats**–No, we don't mean sitting down to a bowl of butter, but there are good fats that help your skin and hair (even nails) look healthier. Try avocados. Just slice one in half and drizzle a little flavored olive oil on it. Nuts and nut butters are great. Once you try almond or cashew butter with a delicious all fruit spread, you'll never go back to peanut butter and jelly!

➤ **Beverages**–We have already talked about water, but let us stress that drinking good, clean water as often as you like is good for the skin. Add a lemon wedge or a slice of your favorite fruit and enjoy a glass of water when you feel an urge to pop open a can of soda–

bad for you and very dehydrating to the skin! We love green tea and white tea, iced or hot, and studies now show that teas are loaded with antioxidants. Your exterior is a reflection of your interior, and your face shows what you are eating. Think about it, when we were teen-agers and ate greasy, fried foods, what happened? Now if we eat a diet depleted of nutrients or if we become dehydrated, our faces will show it by becoming sallow and discolored. And remember, adult acne is a very real thing and can definitely be the result of a diet gone astray and/or a hormonal imbalance.

Tips for Preventing and Eliminating Wrinkles

☆ **Shun the Sun**–Doctors agree that sun exposure accounts for eighty to ninety percent of all skin damage. Knowing that, we should all be using a good sunscreen with at least an SPF of 15 or more. Do not rely on the sunscreen in your make-up. For one thing, it is diluted by the make-up itself and almost never contains a high enough SPF. Do not forget that even on cloudy days a certain amount of ultraviolet ray exposure takes place. We have already discussed the dangers of skin cancer from sun exposure.

☆ **Always wear sunglasses.** They protect your delicate eye area and your irreplaceable sight!

☆ **Quit smoking**–It makes you look old and it kills you. Need we say more?

☆ **Sleep on Your Back**–Have you ever awakened with a big line cut across your face? Sleep in that same position long enough and that line will become a permanent wrinkle. Try sleeping on your back. There are pillows on the market today that will keep you from moving into one of those "wrinkle causing" positions. Sleeping on your back will inhibit "sleep lines" and is actually better for your back and body in general.

Everything we have discussed in the previous pages to benefit your health benefits your skin.

- Drink more water
- Eat more fruits and vegetables
- Rest more
- Eliminate stress
- Exercise often

Look in the mirror and frown. Now, look in the mirror and smile. Isn't it amazing that simply by changing your expression, you can take years off your face? Isn't this just one more good reason to try to keep a joyful and optimistic attitude?

Let's address those wrinkles that are already there.

The good news is that, at long last, there are things you can do not only to prevent new wrinkles but also to get rid of the ones you have already acquired.

In your twenties, the sun may have caused a few wrinkles on your forehead. In your thirties, you may notice that wrinkles have appeared between your eyes. By forty, you are seeing crow's feet; and by the time you are fifty, lines around the nose and mouth have begun to form. The skin loses moisture and elasticity over time, mostly due to a process that begins in our forties when estrogen abates and our connective tissue is reduced.

Recent science has given us many alternatives to aging. The new techniques are amazing and present even more amazing results, but you cannot have unlimited amounts of plastic surgery. Plus, not everyone can afford a plastic surgeon and a facelift. There are other procedures such as dermabrasion and micro-dermabrasion that remove the outer (dead) layer of skin and reveal fresh, new cells beneath. Lasers are offering positive results in the war against wrinkles; and, of course, there are things like collagen and botox injections, chemical peels, even implants. These procedures, however, are not without risks and possible side effects. Maybe you do not want to be that radical.

There are alternatives you can try to improve the texture and elasticity of your skin while getting rid of wrinkles. While the results will be somewhat less dramatic than surgery, they are fairly immediate and often very gratifying. Retin A and alpha-hydroxy acids have earned reputations for smoothing out wrinkles. Although Retin A continues to require a prescription, there are many skin care products that contain alpha hydroxy acids. These acids are derived from wine, milk, apples, lemon, or sugarcane. They will gradually encourage the "peeling off" of the top layers of dead skin and over a period of time will reduce the look of fine lines and wrinkles, including "crow's feet."

There are several non-surgical face-lift kits on the market. You may have seen them on television or read about them in women's magazines.

*We think that our **Miracle Face Lift** is the best available. The **Dee Simmons Miracle Face Lift Kit** contains milk peptides, alpha lipoic acid, and hyaluronic acid in combination with nutrients in a base of aloe vera.*

*The formulation has been shown to reduce lines and wrinkles by 34 percent and enhance skin smoothness by 36 percent in less than one month of regular use. The amazing results from clinical studies show that after only four weeks, skin firmness increases by 67 percent. The **Miracle Face Life Kit** contains several products: the **Miracle Face Lift Powder** and **Activator** that when mixed together and applied to the face and neck produce a tightening, tingling effect, bringing the circulation to the surface; the **Miracle Serum** that contains ingredients designed to "turn back the clock" and is superior to most department store serums for far less cost; the **Miracle Moisturizer** that when applied to the face and neck drenches the skin with natural emollients.*

While a non-surgical face lift cannot possibly produce the same dramatic results as plastic surgery, the results we have seen are remarkable, and people are thrilled with the improvements.

Exfoliate

Think about it. Men's skin looks younger longer even if they are exposed to the sun. Why? It is because they shave everyday. What does that say? Exfoliate.

There are numerous peels, scrubs, and masks on the market that will help to remove old, dead cells on the skin and reveal fresher, younger looking skin beneath. Your skin needs to be clear of dead cells in order to absorb nutrients such as moisturizers, serums, and toners.

Many peels, scrubs, and masks contain abrasive and harmful ingredients such as pecan and walnut hulls and polyethylene (a plastic used to make shampoo bottles, children's toys, even bullet-proof vests). These ingredients can tear the skin and strip its natural pH balance.

Dee Simmons Miracle Peel, formulated with citrus limonium, ananas sativus (pineapple) extract, and our own Green Miracle, is a safe and highly effective way to remove old, dead skin cells and to prepare the skin for the absorption of valuable nutrients such as those contained in our PM Miracle Moisturizer.

- Citrus medica limonium (lemon) extract is a purifying ingredient that reduces the activity of the sebaceous glands that can lead to blemishes, acne, and oily conditions.

- Ananas sativus (pineapple) extract contains bromelain, an enzyme that has a natural exfoliating action on the surface of the skin. It also smooths the skin and reduces surface inflammation.

- Green Miracle is a safe and effective way to remove dead skin cells and to prepare the skin for better absorption of nutrients.

The skin on your body needs to be exfoliated also. In order for your skin to absorb body creams, you need to help it slough off the dead skin cells. There are numerous salt and sugar scrubs on the market that also contain moisturizers. These are good for removing dead skin and softening skin at the same time. We caution you to be careful of slipping when you use these products in the shower or bath.

Daily Skin Care

Skin care is very personal. There are many different skin types and needs. You should develop a daily skin care regimen.

It does not have to be complicated but should include:

> **A good cleanser** or cleansing gel appropriate for your skin type

> **A balancing toner** to regulate the pH balance and to tighten and refresh

> **Moisturizer** to replenish lost moisture and to protect the skin from pollutants and free radicals (substances in our environment that rob our skin and bodies of valuable nutrients and oxygen). Our skin is constantly being dehydrated by the environment. We live in drying conditions with central heat and air. It is important to replenish the lost moisture if you want skin to remain soft and supple.

The **Dee Simmons Skin Care Collection** is formulated to prevent, slow down, and even reverse the signs of aging. Our products are aloe vera based. Aloe provides a superior delivery system to enable your skin to better absorb the valuable nutrients contained in our products.

▷ **Eye cream**–The word to look for in an eye cream is firming. It's that saggy skin around the eyes that is so aging.

Dee Simmons Eye Firming Cream softens fine lines, hydrates, and stimulates the delicate tissue that surrounds the eye. Its unique formulation reduces dark circles and puffiness while repairing, nourishing, and protecting every skin type. Wrinkles will fade as the skin tightens and firms.

AM - Morning Regime:

Step #1: Hydrating Cleanser *for normal to dry skin or* **Cleansing Gel** *for oily skin*

Specially formulated to gently remove surface impurities and makeup while maintaining the skin's natural moisture.

Hydrating Cleanser - *Apply a quarter size amount of cleanser to face and throat using long upward strokes. Leave on for 30 seconds. Remove with warm water.*

Cleansing Gel - *Apply a dime size amount of gel to face and throat using long upward strokes. Leave on for 30 seconds. Remove with warm water.*

Step #2: Balancing Toner *for all skin types*

> *Restores the pH balance of the skin and enhances the penetration of nutrients. Leaves the skin feeling fresh and clean.*

> *Apply a small amount of* **Balancing Toner** *to face and neck with a cotton ball. Gently press into the skin – do not rub.*

Step #3: Miracle Firming Serum *with MiraLift™ Complex for all skin types*

> *Full of amino acids that stimulate fibroblast cells to produce elastin and collagen. Delivers a surge of nutrients to rejuvenate and regenerate facial firmness.*

> *Apply two to three pumps of Miracle Firming Serum to face and neck. Let dry at least one minute before applying moisturizer.*

> *Clinical studies show when using MiraLift™ Complex for 28 days wrinkles decrease by 34%, smoothness is enhanced by 36%, and skin firmness is increased by 67%!*

Step #4: Enriched Moisturizer *for normal to dry skin or* **Oil-Free Moisturizer** *for oily skin*

> *Rich in vitamins, herbs, and humectants that restore moisture balance to the skin.*

> *Apply a quarter size of moisturizer to face and throat using long upward strokes. Wait at least 30 seconds before applying makeup.*

Dee recommends her **Eye Firming Cream** *be used in both the AM and PM regimes. Apply a dime size amount of eye crème by patting gently around the eye area. Safe for use on eyelids.*

- *Diminishes wrinkles and fine lines*
- *Hydrates and firms delicate eye tissue*
- *Reduces dark circles and discolorations*
- *Reduces puffiness*
- *Suitable for all skin types*

PM - Evening Regime:

Step #1: Hydrating Cleanser *for normal to dry skin or* **Cleansing Gel** *for oily skin*

Specially formulated to gently remove surface impurities and makeup while maintaining the skin's natural moisture.

Hydrating Cleanser - *Apply a quarter size amount of cleanser to face and throat using long upward strokes. Leave on for 30 seconds. Remove with warm water.*

Cleansing Gel - *Apply a dime size amount of gel to face and throat using long upward strokes. Leave on for 30 seconds. Remove with warm water.*

Step #2: Balancing Toner *for all skin types*

Restores the pH balance of the skin and enhances the penetration of nutrients. Leaves the skin feeling fresh and clean.

Apply a small amount of **Balancing Toner** *to face and neck with a cotton ball. Gently press into the skin – do not rub.*

Step #3: Miracle Firming Serum *with MiraLift™ Complex for all skin types*

Full of amino acids that stimulate fibroblast cells to produce elastin and collagen. Delivers a surge of nutrients to rejuvenate and regenerate facial firmness.

Apply two to three pumps of Miracle Firming Serum to face and neck. Let dry at least one minute before applying moisturizer.

> *Clinical studies show when using MiraLift™ Complex for 28 days wrinkles decrease by 34%, smoothness is enhanced by 36%, and skin firmness is increased by 67%!*

Step #4: **PM Miracle Moisturizer** *for all skin types*

> *A state of the art advance moisture complex containing hyaluronic acid and alpha lipoic acid for maximum skin hydration. Delivers a heavy dose of moisturizing ingredients deep into the skin to diminish the signs of aging and minimize the appearance of fine lines. Restores moisture balance and pH balance to skin.*
>
> *Apply a quarter size of moisturizer to face and throat using long upward strokes. Leave on overnight.*

Dee recommends her **Eye Firming Cream** *be used in both the AM and PM regimes. Apply a dime size amount of eye crème by patting gently around the eye area. Safe for use on eyelids.*

- *Diminishes wrinkles and fine lines*
- *Hydrates and firms delicate eye tissue*
- *Reduces dark circles and discolorations*
- *Reduces puffiness*
- *Suitable for all skin types*

For aging skin, serums and anti-aging complexes are widely available. Serums containing valuable skin-rejuvenating nutrients have become one of the most popular skin care treatments. Most are quite pricey, but the good ones are also quite effective. Remember when purchasing an anti-aging serum that it is important to see proof of clinical studies.

> *Dee Simmons Miracle Firming Serum* *improves lines and wrinkles by 34 percent, enhances skin smoothness by 36 percent, and increases skin firmness by 67 percent when used as directed over only four weeks.*

There is no substitute for a good daily skin routine.

Hands and Body

One of the first places we show age is our hands. Our hands are constantly exposed to the elements, water, soap, and household chemicals. Try to apply a dab of hand cream every time your hands have been in water. Carry a tube of hand cream in your purse at all times, and do not neglect your cuticles. Rub hand cream into the ends of your fingers. If your hands are exceptionally dry, consider some sleeping gloves to hold the moisture overnight.

A great method of hydrating the skin on your body is to take a warm shower or bath and apply cream while you are still damp. Wrap up in a terry robe until all the moisture has been absorbed into your skin. Try this a few evenings in a row, and you will see a marked difference in your skin's moisture levels.

Don't forget your feet. Apply cream and slip on a pair of old socks until all the cream has been absorbed.

Physical Activity

We have discussed how important exercise is for overall health, but it also benefits the appearance of your skin. It increases circulation that delivers nutrients and allows for a restful sleep which gives the skin the chance to rejuvenate.

Chemical Free is Best

Skin preparations are like food. Just as we recommend organic fruits and vegetables, we also recommend that you select skin products free of chemicals and preservatives.

All **Dee Simmons Skin Care** products are plant-based, natural, and without dangerous chemicals and harmful preservatives that can cause skin irritations or worse.

You will be amazed at how quickly your skin responds to a good, healthy regimen, particularly if it has been neglected. The face in the mirror will thank you!

Remember these tips:

☆ Don't sunbathe. You should always protect your skin from the sun.

☆ If you smoke, stop! Not only is it a cancer causing habit, but it also wrecks your skin by causing the skin's blood vessels to narrow.

☆ Limit alcohol intake–alcohol dehydrates your skin.

☆ Get plenty of rest.

☆ Eat a healthy diet and take good supplements.

☆ Stay hydrated. Drink plenty of water.

☆ Use quality skin care products with proven ingredients.

There is no replacing good health for contributing to your appearance. A healthy, rested person will always look better than someone attempting to maintain a youthful appearance with monthly trips to the dermatologist and frequent trips to the surgeon.

Chapter Seventeen

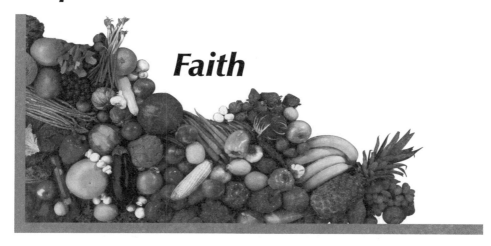

Faith

Current research now supports what many have thought for a very long while, that there is definitely a correlation between good health and spirituality. **Faith is a powerful ally in the war against illness and aging.**

Studies show that spiritual people have less stress, greater life satisfaction, and fewer self-destructive behaviors such as smoking, drinking, and drug abuse. Spirituality has been shown to reduce depression, improve blood pressure, and boost the immune system!

The practice of your religious faith can not only help you heal but, when combined with medical advice and care, can also provide you and your family the greatest opportunity of becoming very healthy.

In 1996, a random survey of 296 members of the American Academy of Family Physicians revealed that ninety-nine percent were "convinced" that religious beliefs can produce better health and healing. An amazing seventy-five percent of those same physicians believe that prayer offered for us by other people has similar effects.

Recent studies by schools of medicine at various universities confirm that the practices of spirituality and religion reduce high blood pressure in women, and researchers are saying that people who regularly attend religious services are twenty-nine percent more likely to live longer than those who do not. Thirty U.S. medical schools now include courses in religion, spirituality, and health in their curricula.

The message is "worship"

Worship is truly individual. If for some reason you are unable to go to church, you may want to watch your favorite service on television; or you may be most comfortable reading your Bible and worshipping privately. Whatever your preference, know that while you are practicing your faith, you are actually improving your health and increasing your longevity.

Religious and spiritual beliefs are an important part of how many people deal with life. As we age, we all know that we begin to face hardships that may not have been factors in our youth. We begin to face the loss of friends and family. Illness is more prevalent as we age. Faith can provide us with the strength to endure hard times as well as giving us a sense of purpose and wonderful guidelines for living a better life. When we face tough situations, including health problems, our religious beliefs and practices can help us fight feelings of helplessness.

Faith and prayer restore meaning and order to life situations that otherwise would seem unbearable. Spirituality promotes a sense of control, and spirituality is an important and powerful source of strength for the faithful.

Medical studies have confirmed that spirituality can have a profound effect on mental states. In a study of men who were hospitalized, nearly half rated religion as helpful in coping with their illness. A second study showed that the more religious patients were, the more quickly they recovered from certain disorders. A third study revealed that high levels of hope and optimism, key factors in fighting depression, were found among those who strictly practiced their religion.

Doctors and scientists once avoided the study of spirituality in connection with medicine, but findings within the past ten years have made many rethink that position. Studies show that religion can help to promote good health and fight disease by offering additional social supports such as religious outreach groups. For someone who has lost a loved one, church and related support groups can be instrumental in helping in grief recovery.

Often life changes such as retirement can be very difficult. Having church and its related activities as a support and outlet can be very rewarding. And, in times of illness, the support, caring, and prayer can make a world of difference both to the patient and his or her caregivers by improving coping skills through prayer and the philosophy that all things have a purpose.

In a seven-year study of older adults, religious faith was associated with less physical disability and less depression. Studies also show that older adults who regularly attend religious services have healthier immune systems than those who do not. They are also more likely to have consistently lower blood pressure. A healthy immune system helps keep us well, and we have learned the ravages of high blood pressure.

Patients undergoing open-heart surgery who received strength and comfort from their faith were three times more likely to survive than those who had no religious ties.

These are confirmed studies performed by traditional medical experts.

When we think about people who remain young, both in appearance and health, they are always those individuals with calm and serene expressions, people who control their stress and practice relaxation. There is no better stress reducer than prayer. Think about it. Prayer is a form of meditation. You are communicating with the Lord; and when you are praying, you are turning your problems and stresses over to Him.

You may already be practicing your faith, but let's take time to assess exactly how. Are you getting up on Sunday morning, hurrying to get dressed, and rushing into the church to be on time after struggling to find a parking place? Do you leave church and immediately run home, throw off your church clothes, and dash to the mall or to do other chores?

On Sundays these days there are many diversions. Shopping malls are open. Grocery stores are open. Discount stores are open. Movies and entertainment centers all remain open on Sundays. We are offered many reasons and lots of excuses for not observing Sunday as intended. In this busy, competitive world, it is easy to let a day of worship and prayer fall behind a day of shopping, yard-work, even football or television. But none of these activities have medical studies that actually prove their positive benefits for our health and longevity.

This week, practice your faith and truly observe the Sabbath. Revel in a day of rest, take time to give thanks, and even more time to reflect on your blessings. I believe that if you let one day be a day of rest and a day of worship, you will find that next week will be happier, more meaningful, and less stressful.

One major component of Sundays years ago was dinner together as a family. These days fast foods and junk foods are far too often part of the "family meal." Let's return Sunday dinner to a real family meal with good, wholesome foods, prayer, and quality time together. It is amazing how problems fall away when compared to the good things in our lives.

Apply these practices to your life. We promise that your health and outlook will improve.

- Attend church regularly and become part of your religious community. You will find worlds of activities on almost any given day or night at your church. We have already discussed the importance of remaining involved as a way to stay young and the positive effects of friendships on our health.

- Focus on your blessings rather than your problems, and offer thanks through prayer often. A positive outlook is a healthy one.

- Plan a day for worship and family. Eliminate unnecessary activities and engage in meaningful time together. Not only will you find yourself relaxing, but the joy you feel will be the release of those healthy endorphins.

- Share good, wholesome meals with friends and family. Stick with God-given natural foods rather than fast, junk foods. God has given us all that we need in nature.

- Face life with faith and optimism.

Chapter Eighteen

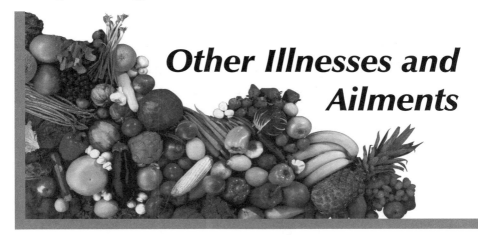

Other Illnesses and Ailments

Alzheimer's Disease–a condition in which nerve cells in the brain die, making it difficult for the brain's signals to be transmitted properly. The death of the nerve cells occurs gradually over a period of years. Common symptoms of Alzheimer's disease include impaired memory and thinking, disorientation and confusion, misplacing things, trouble performing familiar tasks, changes in personality and behavior, poor or decreased judgment, inability to follow directions, problems with language and communication, impaired visual and spatial skills, loss of motivation or initiative, and loss of normal sleep patterns.

There is some connection between Alzheimer's disease and exposure to mercury. Exposure to mercury is routine with dental amalgams. If you still have amalgam fillings, you might consider having them removed and replaced with composite fillings.

Aluminum in deodorants, dandruff shampoo, antacids, and pots and pans has also been associated with Alzheimer's. Do not cook with aluminum cookware, and avoid products that contain aluminum.

Anxiety

Anxiety may include symptoms ranging from rapid heartbeat and hyperventilation to insomnia and high blood pressure. Anxiety can be the result of stress; past experiences; and present pressures such as a divorce, a death in the family, moving, or changing jobs.

If you suffer from anxiety, you should avoid caffeine, sugar, and alcohol. Try foods rich in vitamin C, calcium, and magnesium.

Bladder Infection

Bladder Infection is usually the result of bacteria. Symptoms can include a constant feeling that you need to urinate, difficulty urinating, burning and aching in the bladder region. The urine may have a strong odor and be cloudy. Left untreated, bladder infections can lead to more serious kidney infections.

Try drinking pure cranberry juice (avoid commercial cranberry cocktail loaded with sugar) which acidifies the urine and prohibits bacterial growth. Drink plenty of water. Avoid citrus fruits as they may irritate the bladder. Do not consume alcohol, carbonated beverages, or caffeine. Avoid sugars and spicy foods. If you have pain, sit in a hot bath. Do not "hold" your urine. If you feel the urge to urinate, do so immediately. If the condition persists or if you see blood in your urine, seek medical attention.

Bruising

Bruising occurs when tissues under the skin are damaged. Blood collects resulting in pain, swelling, and discoloration. If you are bruising excessively, you need to see your doctor as bruising without reason can be a sign of serious illness.

People taking aspirin can bruise more easily. Also, people who do not consume enough fresh foods; who smoke; who are overweight, anemic, vitamin C deficient, suffering from leukemia, experiencing excessive menstrual bleeding, or using anti-coagulant drugs may all be susceptible to bruising.

Eat a diet containing plenty of leafy green vegetables and colorful fruits. Bromelain, an enzyme found in pineapple and papaya, is effective in reducing swelling and bruising.

When injured, apply ice immediately to reduce swelling and bruising. Arnica gel is an excellent remedy for bruising.

Burns

Burns–described in degrees: a first degree burn, such as one you would have from touching a hot pan or iron, is characterized by blistering and pain; a second degree burn may have more serious blistering, damaged hair follicles, and scarring; third degree burns are very dangerous and may include damaged and charred flesh as well as tissue and muscle damage, causing the body to lose fluid.

To take the pain out of minor burns, apply ice water or ice immediately. Keep a bottle of aloe vera gel in the refrigerator to dab on minor scrapes and burns. More serious burns require immediate medical attention since burns can cause serious infections.

Colds

Colds–a sign that the immune system is over-taxed (Chapter One). Chicken soup (protein) really works, but do not eat sugary or fried foods, and try to eliminate dairy products. Take in plenty of fluids. Try hot water with lemon (and honey if you must) and fruit juices. Double up on vitamin C.

Eat small meals consisting of plenty of fruits and steamed vegetables.

Some ideas that may help are:

- Sip hot liquids such as chicken broth.

- Flush soiled tissue so you do not re-infect yourself.

- Wash your hands often.

- Be considerate and try not to spread your infection.

- Remain active; don't just lie around. Moving will help to loosen and expel secretions.

Depression

An estimated nineteen million American adults are living with major depression. Depression is characterized by feelings of hopelessness and despair with symptoms including inability to concentrate and lack of enthusiasm. Depressed people may experience physical symptoms such as heart palpitations, headaches, overwhelming fatigue, and weight loss or gain.

To combat depression, eat a diet with plenty of raw fruits and vegetables, soy products, brown rice, millet, and legumes. Complex carbohydrates contain serotonin–a lack of serotonin has been linked to depression. Wheat gluten has been linked to depression so eliminate all wheat products.

Exercise, particularly vigorous exercise, seems to have positive effects on bouts of depression.

Zinc has been found to be deficient in people suffering with depression. Fish oil has been shown to be highly successful in treating depression and related mental illnesses.

Diarrhea

Diarrhea–characterized by loose, watery, and frequent stools often accompanied by cramping. Food allergies are the most common cause of diarrhea. Viruses and bacterial infections can also be culprits.

Drink plenty of liquids. Do not consume dairy products. Avoid alcohol, caffeine, and spicy foods. It is best to let a mild case of diarrhea run its course as it is the body's way of eliminating toxins or bacteria. Stick to a diet of liquids for 24 hours. If diarrhea persists beyond two days, contact your physician. (Chapter 12)

Eating Disorders

Anorexia is a disease characterized by the persons who are affected starving themselves; **bulimia** sufferers binge eat and then purge (vomit). While women are more affected by eating disorders, men periodically suffer from them as well. The pressure to be thin and fit has caused an upsurge of eating disorders.

Persons with an eating disorder may have low blood pressure. They may be irritable or aggressive. Low pulse rate, weakness, dry skin, bad teeth (eroded enamel), halitosis, chronic constipation, even a succession of menstrual periods are all symptoms of eating disorders.

Persons suffering from eating disorders must have professional help to ascertain the root causes of their problems. Once eating patterns are re-established, fresh fruits and vegetables and high protein foods are best. Eliminate sweets and junk foods. Yogurt, whole grain cereals, and protein drinks are helpful to regain weight and nutritional balance.

Flu

Flu (Influenza)–a highly contagious viral infection of the upper respiratory tract. Symptoms begin like those of a cold but come on more quickly and with more severity. Chills and aching with headache and fatigue characterize flu. Flu can be dangerous for older adults and young children or people suffering with chronic illnesses.

Consume plenty of liquids to avoid dehydration. Sleep and rest. Antibiotics are useless in treating viral infections. The best way to avoid catching the flu is to keep out of crowded, closed environments during the flu season, wash your hands frequently, and boost your immune system with good nutrition and supplementation. (Chapter 1)

Hot chicken or turkey soup with a dash of cayenne pepper may help.

Gallstones

Gallstones–formed when cholesterol crystallizes and combines with the bile in the gallbladder. Sometimes a person with gallstones has no symptoms; but if a stone blocks the bile passage, pain in the upper right abdomen accompanied by nausea and vomiting occurs.

During an attack, eat no solid food. Avoid fatty or fried foods. Apple, pear, or beet juice may be helpful. Re-introduce solid foods slowly. Being overweight and obesity are risk factors. (Chapter 13)

Headaches

Headaches–Approximately 45 million Americans suffer from chronic headaches, and of those, 28 million suffer from migraines. Although most headaches are tension-related, other possible causes include allergies; constipation; eyestrain; hunger; sinus pressure; muscle tension; hormonal imbalance; nutritional deficiencies; fever; the use of alcohol, drugs, or tobacco; and exposure to irritants such as pollution, perfumes, dust, or animal dander.

Headaches that occur frequently may be the sign of an underlying problem and should be further investigated.

Eat a well-balanced diet and practice deep-breathing and other relaxation techniques. Get sufficient sleep and rest.

If any of the following symptoms accompany a headache, call your doctor: blurred vision, confusion or loss of speech, fever, stiffness in the neck, sensitivity to light, pressure behind the eyes that is relieved by vomiting, pressure in the facial area behind the sinuses, throbbing in the head and temples, a pounding heart, visual color changes or feeling that your head might explode. Seek medical attention immediately if one of the following occurs: a sudden severe headache like a "thunderclap"; headache after you have had an injury to your head area; headache pain that worsens after coughing, straining, or sudden movement.

Avoid alcohol; caffeine; dairy products; sugar; chocolate; wheat; food containing sulfites, nitrates, and MSG.

For mild headaches try eating turkey to raise serotonin levels, almonds, leafy green vegetables, broccoli, pineapple, and cherries.

Hemorrhoids

Hemorrhoids–enlarged veins that develop in the anal canal. Although uncomfortable at times, this common condition rarely poses a serious problem.

Diets low in fiber and full of refined foods are a cause of hemorrhoids. Other causes are inactivity, not drinking enough water, painkillers, being overweight, obesity, allergies, and pregnancies. Constipation may play a large part in the development of hemorrhoids.

Hemorrhoids can cause itching, pain, and sometimes rectal bleeding. Eat smaller, fiber-rich meals. Taking a teaspoon of olive or flaxseed oil before each meal and drinking plenty of water will help eliminate hemorrhoids. (Chapter 12)

Hepatitis

Hepatitis–inflammation of the liver. There are several types of hepatitis: hepatitus A, known as infectious hepatitis, is spread through person to person contact, blood, or feces. Hepatitus B is a sexually transmitted disease also transmitted through transfused blood, dirty needles, and saliva. Hepatitis C usually follows a blood transfusion with infected blood, sexual contact, or intravenous drug use. Hepatitis D is associated with the Epstein-Barr virus and cytomegalovirus. There are other, less common forms including non-A, non-B, and hepatitis E, all highly contagious.

If you have been diagnosed with hepatitis, drink no alcohol and avoid all fats, sugars, and processed foods. Eat no shellfish, raw fish, or animal protein. Get plenty of rest. Eat plenty of fruits and vegetables including artichokes. Artichokes are excellent liver protectors.

Milk thistle is an excellent supplement for liver support.

***Ultimate Living Immune Support Formula** detoxifies the liver and has been helpful to persons with hepatitis.*

Insomnia

Insomnia–an inability to sleep well. Insomnia is a common problem, affecting almost everyone at one time or another. A person with insomnia may have difficulty falling asleep or staying asleep, may wake up frequently during the night, or may wake up earlier than desired the next morning, resulting in symptoms such as daytime fatigue, irritability, poor memory, loss of productivity, and decreased enjoyment of family and social life.

Avoid alcohol, tobacco, and caffeine. For dinner eat turkey, bananas, figs, dates, yogurt, milk, tuna, and whole grains or nut butters. These foods are high in tryptophan, which promotes sleep.

Avoid chocolate, cheese, bacon, eggplant, ham, potatoes, sauerkraut, sugar, sausage, spinach, tomatoes, and wine before bedtime because they contain tyramine, which increases the release of brain stimulants.

The following are tips that may help you adopt better sleeping patterns:

- Go to bed and awaken at the same time every day.

- Try to start relaxing several hours before bedtime, and never exercise close to bedtime.

- Use the bed for sleep. If you cannot sleep, don't fight the bed; get up.

- Don't drink caffeinated drinks in the evening.

- Do not eat late in the evening.

- Avoid taking any medications late in the day that may act as stimulants, for example, nasal decongestants.

Melatonin is a natural hormone that may help you sleep.

> ***Ultimate Living Cal-Mag Plus*** *can help you relax.*

Jaundice

Jaundice–yellowing of the skin and eyes caused by a buildup of bilirubin (a yellow-brown substance that results from the breakdown of old red blood cells) in the blood. Jaundice is not a disease itself but may be the sign of blood or liver disorders.

Never consume raw or undercooked fish, meat, or poultry. Do not consume any alcohol. Try drinking water with lemon, beet juice, and dandelion or black radish extract, all excellent liver cleansers.

> ***We recommend Ultimate Living Immune Support Formula*** *for blood and liver disorders. We always suggest that you consult your physician before beginning any alternative therapies.*

Kidney Stones

Kidney Stones–accumulations of mineral salts that can lodge in the urinary tract. They can be terribly painful.

For pain relief, try drinking the juice from half a lemon in eight ounces of water every thirty minutes until pain abates. Fresh apple juice is also beneficial. Drink plenty of water. Increase your intake of vitamin A rich fruits and vegetables such as apricots, cantaloupes, carrots, pumpkins, sweet potatoes, and squash. Alfalfa has been used for centuries by the Chinese in the treatment of kidney stones.

Limit your intake of protein and calcium. Use no salt. Avoid colas, all refined sugars, and any foods that lead to the production of oxalic acid. Such foods include asparagus, beets, eggs, fish , parsley, rhubarb, spinach, Swiss chard, and cabbages.

Avoid alcohol, caffeine, chocolate, cocoa, dried figs, nuts, pepper, poppy seeds, and black tea. Exercise.

> *Watercress, an ingredient in* **Ultimate Living Immune Support Formula,** *has been used for centuries to dissolve kidney stones.*

Lyme Disease

Lyme disease (Lyme borreliosis) is a bacterial infection that is spread by ticks. You may develop Lyme disease if you are bitten by an infected tick.

If you find a tick on your body,

- Remove the tick with tweezers, grasping the tick as close to the skin as possible. Do not squeeze the tick as you may cause it to inject bacteria into the skin.

- Thoroughly wash your hands and the bite area. Apply alcohol or a topical antiseptic to the area. Keep the tick in a jar, and take it to your physician to be identified.

- Watch for symptoms for three weeks. Symptoms include small raised bumps or a rash on the skin, fever, chills, nausea, sore throat, and vomiting. Facial paralysis may occur weeks to months later along with enlargement of the spleen, severe headaches, and enlargement of the heart coupled with abnormal heart rhythm. Over the long term, persistent backache, stiff neck, joint pain, and even degenerative muscle disease may result from Lyme disease.

If you suspect that you may have Lyme disease, you must see a physician for proper treatment. Keep you immune system strong by eating plenty of garlic and green foods. (Chapter One)

Motion Sickness

Motion Sickness occurs when motion causes the eyes, the sensory nerves, and the vestibular apparatus of the ear to send conflicting signals to the brain. Anxiety, genetics, overeating, poor ventilation, and traveling immediately after eating are common contributing factors. Symptoms may include headache, queasiness, nausea, vomiting, cold sweats, dizziness, yawning, fatigue and sleepiness, pallor, lack of appetite, and severe distress.

Natural remedies such as charcoal tablets, ginger, magnesium, peppermint, and vitamin B-6 work well for motion sickness.

Try sipping peppermint tea with ginger, or take two ginger capsules (approximately 1,000 milligrams) every three hours, starting one hour prior to travel.

Avoid alcohol; stay cool if possible; limit visual input–in other words, lie down and close your eyes. Breathe deeply through your nose. Do not eat foods likely to upset your stomach when traveling.

Multiple Sclerosis

Multiple sclerosis (MS) affects 2.5 million people worldwide, including 400,000 Americans. It is a progressive, degenerative disorder of the central nervous system, including the brain, the optic nerve, and the spinal cord. Multiple sclerosis comes in flare-ups called exacerbations. Its symptoms vary from person to person depending upon which parts of the brain or spinal cord (central nervous system) are damaged. The loss of myelin and scarring caused by MS can affect any part of the central nervous system.

Symptoms may come and go or become more or less severe from day to day or, rarely, from hour to hour. Symptoms may become more severe with increased (or, less commonly, decreased) body temperature or after a viral infection. Symptoms of MS, such as tremors, pain, and difficulty thinking clearly, are similar to those of many other conditions and do not necessarily mean you have MS.

A strong immune system may help to prevent MS by helping the body avoid infection which often precedes the onset of this disease. (Chapter One)

Eat only organic foods with no preservatives or chemical additives. Eat plenty of raw vegetables and fruits as well as dark leafy greens. Drink plenty of pure water. Never consume alcohol. Take a good fiber supplement.

Supplements such as CoQ10, Omega-3 fatty acids, garlic, vitamin B complex, and choline are all helpful.

Pancreatitis

Pancreatitis– inflammation of the pancreas, a gland that lies behind the stomach. The pancreas produces the hormones insulin and glucagon to control metabolism. It also produces other hormones and enzymes that aid in the digestion of fats, proteins, and carbohydrates. The hormones and enzymes flow from the pancreas through the pancreatic duct into the upper part of the small intestine (duodenum).

Inflammation occurs when these digestive enzymes leak out of the pancreatic duct and attack the pancreas. The inflammation may develop suddenly (acute pancreatitis) or over many years (chronic pancreatitis). Pancreatitis causes severe pain in the area of the navel and radiating to the back. The pain is typically worsened by movement and may be accompanied with nausea and vomiting, sometimes severe. Other symptoms include upper abdominal swelling and distention; excessive gas; fever; sweating; hypertension; muscle aches; and abnormal, fatty stools.

If you have symptoms of pancreatitis, call your physician. This is an extremely serious condition that requires medical attention.

Eat a diet low in fat and sugar. Consume NO alcohol.

Parkinson's Disease

Parkinson's disease is diagnosed in more than 50,000 Americans each year. It is a degenerative disease affecting the nervous system. The underlying cause is yet unknown, but symptoms appear when there is a lack of dopamine in the brain. Dopamine is a neurotransmitter that carries messages from one nerve cell to another.

The disease may start with a mild to moderate tremor of the hand or hands while at rest, a general slow and heavy feeling, muscular stiffness, and a tendency to tire more easily than is normal.

Parkinson's affects men more than women.

Vitamins C and E as well as selenium are essential for Parkinson's patients. Since it is imperative that the person limit toxins in the body, organic foods with no chemicals or preservatives are essential. Ginkgo biloba may help to improve memory and brain functions.

Pneumonia

Pneumonia–a serious infection of the lungs caused by viruses, bacteria, fungi, and microscopic organisms. The infection causes the tiny air sacs in the lungs to become inflamed and to fill with mucus, even pus.

Symptoms can include fever, chills, cough, bloody sputum, muscle aching, fatigue, sore throat, enlarged lymph glands, a bluish cast to the skin and nails, pain in the chest, and difficult, rapid respiration (breathing).

Pneumonia is typically preceded by an upper respiratory infection such as a cold, influenza, or measles. Factors that increase the risk of pneumonia include aspiration under anesthesia; being over sixty years old; having a weakened immune system, cardiovascular disease, diabetes, HIV infection, a seizure or stroke, kidney failure, sickle cell disease, malnutrition, and even allergies. Alcoholism, smoking, foreign bodies in the respiratory passages, and exposure to chemical irritants are also contributing factors. A positive diagnosis can only be made with a chest x-ray.

See your health-care provider if your suspect pneumonia. Pneumonia is potentially dangerous.

Vitamins A and C plus bioflavonoids are essential. Drink plenty of fresh juices. Liquids help to thin lung secretions. Drink plenty of water with lemon slices. DO NOT SMOKE!

Rheumatic Fever

Rheumatic Fever–a condition primarily affecting children that usually follows a strep infection. Symptoms include skin rash, shortness of breath, sore throat, poor circulation, fever, and extreme fatigue. Arthritis is the most common symptom and may last a lifetime.

Avoid sugar, refined foods, fried foods, and caffeine. Drink plenty of pure water as well as fruit and vegetable juices.

Shingles

Shingles (herpes zoster) is a viral infection of the nerve roots. It causes pain and a band of rash that spreads on one side of your body. Shingles is caused by the same virus that causes chicken pox. Once you've had chicken pox, the virus lies dormant (inactive) in your nerve roots. If it becomes active again, it causes shingles, not another case of chicken pox.

The virus can be reactivated when the immune system is weakened, so the best prevention for shingles is a strong immune system (Chapter One). It is important to keep stress to a minimum as stress is known to trigger an outbreak of shingles.

> ***Ultimate Living B Complex-Lingual*** *is helpful in the treatment of shingles.*

Tuberculosis

Tuberculosis (TB)–a bacterial infection that usually affects the lungs but can affect other parts of the body such as the bones, kidney, spleen, intestines, and liver. Tuberculosis is highly contagious and is found throughout the world. It had been nearly eradicated in the U.S.; but with the rise of global travel, AIDS, and drug use, tuberculosis now appears more frequently than it has in previous decades.

Symptoms of TB may be slow in developing and often resemble those of the flu: general malaise, coughing, night sweats, loss of appetite, chest pain, and low-grade fever. As the condition worsens, increasing amounts of sputum are produced with increased night sweats, fever, weight-loss, and shortness of breath. Blood may also appear in the sputum.

Unlike most infectious illnesses, TB is chronic.

A strong supplement program is essential in fighting tuberculosis as opportunistic infections can be a problem.

Dee and D'Andra's Ten Tips for Healthy Living

1. *Get up and move!*

We have already drawn the connection between staying healthy and getting plenty of physical activity. Exercise and physical activity improve your energy levels, boost your immune system, and give you a brighter outlook. Find an activity you enjoy and start today.

2. *Eat a healthy diet!*

Cut down on fats and sweets. Eat more fruits and vegetables, more whole grains, and cold-water fish instead of red meat. Try green foods–they are full of nutrients and valuable substances for your health.

3. *Avoid chemicals, pesticides, and preservatives. Do not use artificial sweeteners.*

Aspartame–The popularity of sugar-free foods and drinks has escalated with America's obsession with weight loss. Aspartame is about 200 times sweeter than sugar, so smaller amounts of it are necessary to produce sweetness. Aspartame has been linked with a variety of health problems, not the least of which are headaches, mood swings, vision problems, nausea and diarrhea, sleep disorders, memory loss, confusion, and convulsions (in some people with allergic reactions).

Try stevia, a natural plant-based sweetener with similar sweetening capacity to aspartame and none of the dangers. Stevia is readily available at your health food store or at grocery stores that carry natural foods. It comes in liquid or powder–even convenient packets to carry in your pocket or purse.

4. *Take good, quality supplements.*

Our diets today require that we bridge the nutrition gap by taking good supplements. Adequate nutrition is essential in keeping our immune systems strong and our bodies healthy.

5. *Relax.*

It is important for your body to relax. You can do so in any number of ways. Meditation, deep breathing, and even reading can all provide ways for you to take it easy. Better yet, take a pleasant walk, and you will shed pounds along with stress.

6. *Watch your weight.*

It is a matter of health, not vanity. If you have too much fat, particularly around the waist area, you are at a higher risk for a number of additional health problems, such as diabetes, heart disease, and stroke. Avoid overloading on carbohydrates, sweets, and fatty foods.

7. *Floss your teeth.*

Recent studies make a direct connection between longevity and teeth flossing. Nobody knows exactly why. Perhaps it is because people who floss tend to be more health conscious than people who don't. Thought for the day: Floss and be your body's boss.

FYI: Your dentist should always be made aware of any special health conditions or any medications you are taking.

8. *Keep a positive mental outlook.*

There is a definite connection between living well and healthfully and having a cheerful outlook on life.

9. *Protect yourself from pollution.*

If you can't live in a smog-free environment, at least avoid smoke-filled rooms, high traffic areas, breathing in highway fumes, and exercising near busy thoroughfares. Exercise outside when the smog rating is low. Exercise indoors in air conditioning when air quality is poor. Plant shrubbery in your yard; it is a good deterrent against pollution and dirt from the street.

Good supplements help the body resist the effects of pollution.

10. *Practice your faith.*

Faith provides you the strength to face physical and emotional challenges.

> *And please do not undo all the good advice we have provided by smoking, consuming too much alcohol, or not wearing your seat belt.*

Ultimate Living International
3131 Turtle Creek Blvd. Suite # 510
Dallas, Texas 75219
(214) 220-1240

Ordering Information:
1-800-360-0988 or www.deesimmons.com

Founded in 1996 by cancer survivor Dee Simmons, Ultimate Living International's mission is to provide the highest quality nutritional supplements and skin care products available on the market today, and to offer the most current information on health and wellness issues to the consumer. Through intensive research, relationships with world renowned physicians and clinicians, and meticulous product formulation and analysis, Ultimate Living products are manufactured according to the highest pharmaceutical standards and are formulated to strengthen the immune system, fight debilitating degenerative illness, and assist in the healing process when illness occurs. With dedication to the well-being of our customers, our associates, and the environment, every effort to attain the utmost purity and highest quality is made in the production of Ultimate Living's family of all-natural or organically grown nutritional supplements and skin care products.

As you have found through reading the previous pages, there is power in green. The foundation of our product line is Green Miracle. Green Miracle has been described as a "health food store in a can" and was specifically developed to fight disease by strengthening the immune system and to provide the daily requirements of fruits, vegetables, and other valuable nutrients. Each and every Ultimate Living product is formulated to provide you with everything you need to meet your body's nutritional needs.

You can trust in the purity and efficacy of our supplement products and in the purity, reliability, and cutting-edge effects of our skin care products.

At Ultimate Living, we work tirelessly to keep you looking and feeling your best!

Ultimate Living Supplements *are formulated with the highest quality, purest ingredients available. They contain no preservatives or harmful chemicals of any kind. All are pharmaceutical grade prepared under the strictest standards. You can order Ultimate Living products with the confidence that you are doing the very best for your health!*

Ultimate Living Green Miracle

"A Health Food Store in a Can"

Three scoops of Green Miracle provide 8,000 mgs of pure nutrition plus your total daily requirement of fruits and vegetables. Green Miracle contains essential vitamins, minerals, amino acids, lignans, chlorophyll, and enzymes. It also assists in regulating the body's pH balance, helps to maintain proper glucose levels, stabilizes the metabolism, provides much needed energy, and gives a powerful boost to your immune system.

Ultimate Living Aloe-Papaya

Ultimate Living Aloe-Papaya is the best tasting aloe drink on the market. Aloe-Papaya is a delicious combination of all organically grown juices certified for purity by the International Aloe Science Council.

Ultimate Living Ionic Trace Minerals

Ultimate Living Ionic Trace Minerals provide over 50 minerals in nature's perfect balance. The source for Ultimate Living minerals is The Great Salt Lake with the highest known concentration of minerals existing in a perfect pH balance. Our minerals are 99.5% sodium free and are 26 times more concentrated than colloidal minerals. Ionic Trace Minerals replace minerals missing from the average diet.

Ultimate Living Immune Support Formula

Ultimate Living Immune Support Formula is our proprietary blend of herbs carefully processed to maintain 100% of the integrity of each ingredient. As a result, Ultimate Living Immune Support Formula releases all the medicinal properties to provide powerful immune-strengthening benefits. Immune Support Formula is an effective blood cleanser and purifier. It also aids in liver cleansing, helps with sugar cravings, and may help with recurrences of auto-immune and inflammatory disorders.

Ultimate Living Multi-Vitamin

Ultimate Living Multi-Vitamin contains over 40 valuable nutrients. Plus, our potent Multi-Vitamin contains 400 IU's of pure vitamin E. Ultimate Living Multi-Vitamin 4 Kids is a great way to give your children the perfect nutritional head-start.

Ultimate Living Men's Formula

Ultimate Living Men's Formula helps promote good prostate health and urinary function and may help to regulate cholesterol and blood pressure.

Ultimate Living Cal-Mag Plus

Ultimate Living Cal-Mag Plus is a superior formula containing Hydroxyapatite, the most absorbable form of calcium. It assists in preventing bone loss and provides nutritional support for tendon, nerve, and muscle tissue.

Ultimate Living Complete Hormone Program

Ultimate Living Complete Hormone Program contains Harmony Cream, an easy to apply pharmaceutical grade progesterone cream (wild yam) providing natural relief from menopausal and PMS symptoms,as well as Hormone Balance capsules specifically designed to provide relief from menopausal symptoms.

Ultimate Living Natural Deodorant

Ultimate Living Natural Deodorant is an exclusive blend of organic, natural based ingredients and contains no aluminum or propylene glycol.

Ultimate Living Cardio Care

Ultimate Living Cardio Care is nutritional support for cardiovascular function. It supports coronary vessel function and circulation while assisting in lowering blood pressure and cholesterol levels.

Ultimate Living CoQ10

Ultimate Living CoQ10 is three times more bioavailable than ordinary CoQ10. The body assimilates it quickly and efficiently. Ultimate Living CoQ10 provides much needed energy to the heart muscle for optimum performance.

Ultimate Living Arthritis Formula

Ultimate Living Arthritis Formula provides nutritional support to revitalize aging cartilage and ease joint pain while providing healing lubrication.

Ultimate Living Super Green Miracle Relief Gel

Ultimate Living Super Green Miracle Relief Gel offers instant penetrating relief from pain and joint inflammation, soothes muscle soreness, and increases blood flow to joints to restore flexibility.

Ultimate Living Lung Formula

Ultimate Living Lung Formula aids in alleviating bronchial spasms, wheezing, and coughing. Respiratory problems such as dry cough and lung and sinus congestion respond positively to Ultimate Living Lung Formula's effective combination of vitamins, minerals, and herbs.

Ultimate Living Weight Loss

Ultimate Living Weight Loss formula will safely help you lose unwanted pounds without harmful or dangerous ingredients. Combined with sensible eating and exercise, you will see dramatic weight loss results and a return of energy and vitality.

Ultimate Living Complete Enzymes

Ultimate Living Complete Enzymes help to keep your digestive tract healthy and functioning properly while aiding in the breakdown of carbohydrates, fat, protein, and fiber. Ultimate Living Complete Enzymes also provide relief from heartburn, indigestion and acid reflux.

Ultimate Living Fiber Cleanse

Ultimate Living Fiber Cleanse is a gentle 15 day digestive cleanser used four times per year to eliminate the build-up of toxins while promoting overall digestive health.

Ultimate Living B-Complex Lingual

Ultimate Living B-Complex Lingual assists in lowering elevated homocysteine levels while painlessly delivering as much B-12 as an injection. Two B-Complex Lingual tablets daily deliver all the required B-vitamin needs as well as the perfect amount of folic acid for women of childbearing age.

Ultimate Living Super Antioxidant

Ultimate Living Super Antioxidant is fifty times more potent than vitamin C and 20 times more potent than vitamin E. Super Antioxidant can help your immune system battle the constant barrage of free radicals.

Ultimate Living Green Miracle for Pets

Ultimate Living Green Miracle for Pets is a complete nutritional supplement for your pets. Green Miracle for Pets promotes healthy heart function, good circulation, and strong muscles and joints while contributing to healthy skin and a shiny coat.

The Dee Simmons Skin Care line is formulated with the same care and pride we dedicate to our supplements. We stay on the leading edge of anti-aging presenting the most effective products available. Our skin care products are all natural, plant-based formulations to help you maintain or regain that youthful appearance.

Dee Simmons Miracle Peel Kit

Dee Simmons Miracle Peel Kit gently exfoliates even sensitive skin without the use of harsh, abrasive chemicals or acids. The plant-based formula effectively removes dry, coarse, dead skin cells and deep pore impurities to reveal fresh, glowing skin.

Dee Simmons Miracle Face Lift Kit

Dee Simmons Miracle Face Lift Kit stops the signs of aging and produces a younger look instantly without the side effects of medical procedures or the downtime of surgery. The easy three step application takes only half an hour in the privacy of your own home.

Dee Simmons Eye Firming Cream

Dee Simmons Eye Firming Cream diminishes wrinkles and fine lines, reduces puffiness, hydrates and firms delicate eye tissue, and reduces dark circles and discolorations.

Dee Simmons Miracle Firming Serum

Dee Simmons Miracle Firming Serum is backed by clinical studies showing a 34% reduction in wrinkles, a 36% enhancement of skin smoothness, and an amazing 67% improvement in skin firmness after only four weeks of use.

Dee Simmons Wrinkle Control Oil

Dee Simmons Wrinkle Control Oil reduces the visible signs of aging and minimizes wrinkles while nourishing the skin with potent antioxidants, essential fatty acids, and vitamins.

Dee Simmons Daily Skin Care Collections

Dee Simmons Daily Skin Care Collections for Normal to Dry or Oily Skin provide the perfect daily skin care regimen for your specific skin type.

Dee Simmons PM Moisturizer

Dee Simmons PM Moisturizer with hyaluronic and alpha lipoic acids repairs the skin while you sleep fighting wrinkles and eliminating the signs of aging.

Dee Simmons Ultimate Shampoo and Conditioner

Dee Simmons Ultimate Shampoo and Conditioner are gentle formulas for all hair types to add sheen, volume and silky softness.

Dee Simmons Green Tea Shower and Bath Gel

Dee Simmons Green Tea Shower and Bath Gel refreshes and soothes skin without irritating or drying with a delightful fresh scent.

Dee Simmons Hand and Body Cream

Dee Simmons Hand and Body Cream is a rich, nourishing blend of vitamins, minerals, antioxidants, and soothing herbs to restore moisture to even the driest skin.

References and Suggested Reading

Books

These books offer excellent information on health and nutrition.

Adderly, Brenda, M.H.A., with Lisa De Angelis, M.S., C.C.P. *The Arthritis Cure Cook Book*. Washington, D.C.: Lifeline Press, 1998.

Balch, James F., M.D., and Phyllis A. Balch, C.N.C. *Prescription for Nutritional Healing*. Garden City Park, New York: Avery Publishing Group, 1997.

Broer, Ted. *Maximum Energy*. Lake Mary, Florida: Creation House, 1999.

Cherry, Reginald, M.D. *The Doctor and the Word*. Orlando, Florida: Creation House, 1996.

Contreras, Francisco, M.D. *A Tomato a Day*. San Diego, California: Interpacific Press, 2002.

Maccaro, Janet, Ph.D., C.N.C. *Natural Health Remedies*. Love Mary, Florida: Siloam, A Strang Company, 2003.

Marangu, Makena, M.D., and Dee Simmons. *Face to Face*. Dallas, Texas: Dee Simmons and Dr. Makena Marangu, 2004.

Marti, James E. *The Alternative Health and Medicine Encyclopedia*. Detroit, Michigan: Visible Ink Press, 1995.

Nelson, Miriam E., Ph.D. *Strong Women, Strong Bones*. New York City, New York: G.P. Putnam's Sons, 2000.

Null, Gary, Ph.D. *Ultimate Anti-Aging Program*. New York City, New York: Kensington Publishing Corp., 1999.

Quillin, Patrick, Ph.D., R.D., C.N.S. *Beating Cancer with Nutrition.* Tulsa, Oklahoma: Nutrition Times Press, 1997.

Rivera, Hugo, and James Villepigue. *The Body Sculpting Bible for Men.* Long Island, New York: Hatherleigh Press/Getfitnow.com Books, 2004.

Salaman, Maureen. *The Cancer Answer.* Menlo Park, California: Statford Publishing, 1984.

Salaman, Maureen. *Foods that Heal.* Menlo Park, California: Statford Press, 1989.

Simmons, Dee. *7 Days to Feeling Better and Looking Younger.* Mansfield, Ohio: BookMasters, Inc. 2003.

Simmons, Dee. *Surviving Cancer.* Tulsa, Oklahoma: Harrison House, 2001.

Simmons, *Dee. Ultimate Living.* Lake Mary, Florida: Siloam Press, 1999.

Sinatra, Stephen T., M.D. *Optimum Health.* New York City, New York: Bantam Books, 1997.

Smith, Pamela, R.O. *Healthy Expectations.* Lake Mary, Florida: Creation House, 1998.

Periodicals

Anderson-Parrado, Patricia. "The Road to Long-term Weight Loss may not be Short, but it is Safe." *Better Nutrition Magazine.* January 1998, pp 22-24.

Alberto, Susanne. "What Women Need: The Latest Breast Health Updates." *Health Products Business Magazine.* October 2001, pp 30-33.

Resources

"Biblical Prescription for Menopause." *Living Healthy and Whole, Christian Broadcasting Network.* 2002.

Block, Will. "Galantamine Helps Keep your Mind on the Money: Memory and Cognitive Impairment can be Costly in more Ways than One." *Life Enhancement.* July 2003, pp 4-8.

Block, Will. "Mastic Kills the Bugs that Cause Gastritis and Ulcers." *Life Enhancement.* July 2003, pp 30-31.

Borek, Carmia, Ph.D. "Weight Loss is about Gaining Control." *Better Nutrition Magazine.* June 1998, pp 22-26.

"Calcium, Magnesium, and Aging." *Women's Health Letter.* Volume 7, pp 1-4.

Contreras, Victor, M.D. "Antioxidant Breakthrough." *Journal of Longevity.* Volume 5, Number 3, pp 28-31.

Dolby, Victoria. "U.S. Diet Shows Small Improvement, but Most Choose Pizza over Veggies." *Better Nutrition Magazine.* November 1996, p 14.

Doss, Larry, M.D. "How to Manage Food Cravings: The Key to Dieting Success." *Journal of Longevity.* 2001, Volume 7, Number 12, pp 34-36.

Engleman, Laura. "Children's Supplements." *Health Supplement Retailer.* January 1996, pp 28-30.

Gazetta, Karolyn A. "Nutritional Supplements for Kids." *Health Counselor.* Volume 8, No.2, pp 31-32.

Ghaly, Fouad I., M.D. "Colon Health for a Healthier You." *Life Solutions.* 2000, p 9.

Gorman, Christine. "Why so Many of us are Getting Diabetes." *Time Magazine.* 8 December 2003, pp 58-69.

Handley, Rich. "Natural Health for Today's Man." *Health Products Business Magazine.* June 2003, pp 12-18.

Handley, Rich. "Taking the Stress out of Stress Relief." *Health Products Business Magazine.* December 2002, pp 28-37.

"Healthbites." *Better Nutrition Magazine.* January 1998, p 12.

Holmes, Steve, and Mark Olsen, M.Sc. "Specialty Supplements, Drug-Free Solutions to Attention Deficit Disorder (ADD)." *Health Supplement Retailer.* December 1997, pp 42-43.

Langer, Stephen, M.D. "Cancer and Nutritional Approaches to Health." *Better Nutrition Magazine.* January 1998, pp 32-46.

Langer, Stephen, M.D. "Colds and Flu are Nothing to Sneeze at." *Better Nutrition Magazine.* November 1996, pp 54-63.

Langer, Stephen, M.D., and James J. Gormley. "Living Longer, Living Better." *Better Nutrition Magazine.* June 1998, pp 44-48.

Lawrence, Ronald M., M.D., Ph.D. "Fat in the Diet: How to Attain the Good Fats and Avoid the Bad." *Health Products Business Magazine.* February 2001, pp 50-56.

Lieskovan, Edward M., Pharm.D. "Prostate Disease–The Facts and Proactive Solutions." *Life Solutions Magazine.* 2000, pp 5-8.

Marchetti, Domenica. "What's your Craving?" *Cooking Light.* November 2001.

Resources

Miller, Cara. "Guide to Getting Fit." *Health Supplement Retailer.* February 1996, pp 22-34.

Millar, Heather. "New Hope in the Treatment of Prostate Cancer." *Spirit Magazine.* 2000, pp 54-143.

"Nutrition and Your Health." *Pathway to Healing.* July/August 1999, pp 6-7.

O'Neil, Joelle, D.O. "New Therapies to Combat Cardiovascular Disease." *Life Solutions.* 2000, p 14-16.

Penrice, John W. "A History of ADD." ADD *News for Christian Families.* July/August 1996.

Picaro, Massimo, M.D. "The Metabolic Approach to Health and Well-being." *Health Supplement Retailer.* January 2001, p 58.

"Poor Nutrition Linked in Elderly to Increased Meds." *Natural Products Industry Insider.* May 2001, p 43.

"Preventing Colon Cancer." *Health Counselor.* Volume 8, Number 2.

Schiavetta, Michael. "Diabetes on the Rise." *Health Products Business Magazine.* August 2003, pp 20-24.

Schulze, Richard, M.D. "Get Well! For Men Only" *Dr. Schulze Bi-Monthly Newsletter.* July 2001, pp 15-22.

Schulze, Richard, M.D. "Get Well! For Women Only" *Dr. Schulze Bi-Monthly Newsletter.* July 2001, pp 5-13.

Simmons, D'Andra. "Revisiting Hormone Replacement Therapy." *Health and Wellness Quarterly.* Volume 6, Issue 4, pp 4-5.

Smith, Nancy. "Good Carbohydrates–Bad Carbohydrates." *Today's Dallas Woman.* March 2001, p 40.

Spock, Benjamin, M.D. "Good Nutrition for Kids." *Physicians Committee for Responsible Medicine.* Spring/Summer 1998, Volume 7, Number 21.

"Tips for a Healthy Heart." *Heart Healthy, A Publication of Medical City Heart.* 2004.

"Tomatoes May Protect Against Cancer." *Health Products Business Magazine.* June 1999, p 48.

Whitaker, Julian, M.D. "Boost Immunity." *Health and Healing.* March 1998, Volume 8, Number 3, p 3.

Whitaker, Julian, M.D. "The Smoking Gun in Heart Disease and Stroke." *Health and Healing.* August 1997.

Williams, David, M.D. "FACT: Over 50% of Today's Health Advice is Wrong and Obsolete!" *Alternatives for the Health Conscious Individual.* Fall 2004, pp 4-6.

Wolfson, David, N.D. "Solving Sinusitis." *Nutrition Science News.* April 2000, pp 158-162.

Woods, Patricia. "Slim Solutions for Summer: Natural Weight Loss Products to the Rescue." *Health Products Business.* May 2003, pp 16-20.

Websites

"ADD/ADHD." *Remedyfind.* http://remedyfind.com/hc-ADD-ADHD.asp (February 7, 2005).

"Allergies: Vitamin C." *About.com.* http://allergies.about.com/od/vitaminc/ (February 9, 2005).

Altshul, Sara. "Cinnamon: The Spice that Cuts Cholesterol and Blood Sugar." *Prevention.com.* http://www.prevention.com/article/0,5778,s1-1-52-160-3974-1,00.html (February 23, 2005).

"Antioxidant Vitamins." *American Heart Association.* http://www.americanheart.org/presenter.jhtml?identifier=4452 (February 15, 2005).

"Cancer and Vitamin C." *Cforyourself.* http://www.cforyourself.com/Conditions/Cancer/cancer.html (March 1, 2005).

"Children's Nutrition Guide." *About.com.* http://pediatrics.about.com/gi/dynamic/offsite.htm?zi=1/XJ&sdn=pediatrics&zu=http%3A%2F%2Fwww.keepkidshealthy.com%2Fnutrition%2F (January 25, 2005).

"Chronic Bronchitis." *The Lung Association.* http://www.lung.ca/diseases/chronic_bronchitis.html (February 1, 2005).

"Chronic Obstructive Pulmonary Disease." *About.com* http://adam.about.com/reports/000070_10.htm (January 19, 2005).

"Chronic Obstructive Pulmonary Disease." *WebMD.* http://aolsvc.health.webmd.aol.com/hw/health_guide_atoz/hw32561.asp (February 7, 2005).

"Diabetes and Cardiovascular(Heart) Disease." American Diabetes Association. http://www.diabetes.org/diabetes-statistics/heart-disease.jsp (February 22, 2005).

"The Diabetic Diet." *Diabetes Information Library.* http://www.diabetessymptom.net/news/news_item.cfm?NewsID=50 (March 1, 2005).

"Exercise Benefits People with Lung Disease." *American Lung Association of California.* http://www.californialung.org/spotlight/03fw_exercise.html (January 19, 2005).

"Feeding Your Immune System." *AskDrSears.com.* http://www.askdrsears. com/html/4/t042500.asp (March 1, 2005).

"Fitness for Specific Health Conditions." *WebHealthCenter.com.* http://www. webhealthcentre.com/general/ft_health.asp#diabetes. (February 9, 2005).

"General Information on Breast Cancer." *Imaginis, The Breast Health Resource.* http://imaginis.com/breasthealth/ (March 1, 2005).

"High Blood Pressure." *HeartCenterOnline.* http://www.heartcenteronline. com/myheartdr/common/articles.cfm?ARTID=365 (February 22, 2005)

"High Levels of Vitamin E Cut Prostate Cancer Risk." http://www.nlm.nih. gov/medlineplus/news/fullstory_23307.html (February 18, 2005).

"Information about Diabetes." *Diabetes Information Library.* http://www. diabetessymptom.net/news/news_item.cfm?NewsID=50 (March 1, 2005).

"Isoflavones." *Isofavones.Info.* http://www.isoflavones.info/ (February 2, 2005).

"Ketones and Diabetes." *Diabetes Now.* http://www.diabetesnow.co.uk/library/ ketones.asp (February 9, 2005).

"Men's Health." *Health Bulletin–Using Foods Instead of Drugs for Health.* http://www.healthbulletin.org/mens_health/men6.htm (February 28, 2005).

Resources

"Nutrition and Breast Health." *University of Virginia Health Care System.* http://www.healthsystem.virginia.edu/internet/cancer/nutrition-breast.cfm (January 29, 2005).

"Parenting Tips." *Friends Hospital.com.* http://www.friendshospitalonline. org/parenting%20tips.html (February 18, 2005).

"Perimenopause." *Bloomingtonwebguide.* http://www.bloomingtonwebguide. com/perimeno.htm (February 18, 2005).

"Product Review: Coenzyme Q10." *ConsumerLab.com.* http://www. consumerlab.com/results/CoQ10.asp (February 10, 2005).

"Prostate Cancer Information Center." *Infoaging.org.* http://www.infoaging. org/d-prost-17-r-selenium.htm (February 4, 2005).

"Prostate Cancer." *Henry Ford Health System.* http://www.henryford.com/ body.cfm?id=41159#screening
(January 26, 2005).

The Role of Diet in the Prevention of Prostate Cancer." *The Prostate Cancer Charity.* http://www.prostatecancer.org.uk/learn/prostateCancer/prevention/ diet.asp (February 1, 2005).

"Social Support: A Buffer against Life's Ills." CNN.com. http://www.cnn.com/ HEALTH/library/MH/00041.html
(February 15, 2005).

Strum, Stephen B., M.D. "Vitamin E." *Prostate Cancer Research Institute PCRI.* http://www.prostate-cancer.org/education/nutrprod/vite.html (February 19, 2005).

"2002 Heart and Stroke Statistical Update." *American Heart Association, American Stroke Association.* http://www.americanheart.org/downloadable/ heart/1014832809466101319090123HS_State_02.pdf (February 4, 2005).

Tybulewicz, Victor L.J. "The Immune System in Health and Disease." *MRC/National Institute for Medical Research.* http://www.nimr.mrc.ac.uk/ MillHillEssays/2000/immunology.htm (January 28, 2005).

"Types of Arthritis." *The Arthritis Society.* http://www.arthritis.ca/ types%20of%20arthritis/default.asp?s=1 (February 20, 2005).

"Ways to Strengthen the Immune System." *PageWise.* http://kyky.essortment. com/immunesystemst_rzzb.htm (February 9, 2005)

"Who Gets Diabetes?" *dLife.* http://www.dlife.com/dLife/do/ShowContent/ about_diabetes/who_gets_diabetes/index.html (February 10, 2005)